GOLF NUTRITION

Filippo Scalise

"When talented, motivated and highly trained athletes meet for competition the margin between victory and defeat is usually small. When everything else is equal, nutrition can make the difference between winning and losing"

(Prof.Ronald John Maughan, St Andrews University, St Andrews, UK)

TABLE OF CONTENTS

Introduction ……………………………………………………………… Pag. 4

1. The energy expenditure of a golf player …………………………… Pag. 7
   - The sample case …………………………………………….. Pag. 9
2. Evaluation of the nutritional status and body composition …………..…. Pag. 12
3. Macronutrients …………………………………………………. Pag. 16
   - Carbohydrates …………………………………………… Pag. 16
   - Proteins ……………………………………………….. Pag. 18
   - Fats ……………………………………………………… Pag. 19
   - The sample case ………………………………………… Pag. 20
4. Micronutrients ……………………………..…………………….. Pag. 22
5. Nutrition for golf ………...………………………………………. Pag. 23
   - The training session …………………………………….. Pag. 24
   - The pre-competition session …………………………….. Pag. 26
   - The competition session ………………………………… Pag. 28
   - The post competition session …………………………… Pag. 29
6. Hydration ……………………………………………………….. Pag. 31
   - Pre-competition hydration ...……………………………… Pag. 32
   - Hydration during the competition ………………………… Pag. 34
   - Post competition hydration ………………...……………… Pag. 35
7. Nutritional aspects linked to sleep and travel ……………………….. Pag. 37
8. Vegetarian diet …………………………………………………… Pag. 41
   - Supplements in the vegetarian diet …...…………………… Pag. 43
   - Creatine ……………………………………………….. Pag. 43
   - Iron ……………………………………………………… Pag. 44
   - Vitamins …………………………………………………. Pag. 44
9. Vegan diet ……………………………………………………… Pag. 45
10. Supplements ..…………………………………………………… Pag. 48
   - Caffeine…………………………………………………... Pag. 49

- Antioxidants .... Pag. 51
- Probiotics .... Pag. 52

11. Supplement 1: nutrion plans.................................... Pag. 57

12. Supplement 2: golf player nutritional questionnaire .... Pag. 60

13. Bibliography .... Pag. 62

Introduction

Golf is a very old sport, which you can play either at an amateur level or at a pro level, in circuits around the world. During 2019 PGA Tour, Brooks Koepla leaded the average score of the season with 69.3 shots, thus winning 9,684,006 USD. However, Charley Hoffman closed it at 141st place in the money list with an average score of 71.3 (only 2 more shots!), gaining 1,468,855 USD.

With such low margins, golf players have always been looking for every possible way to realize the best scores.

Physical endurance and mental concentration are key to improve every shot, but at the same time are hard to keep all along the competition. Despite hard training and ground-breaking equipment, pros know too well that results often come from minimal advantages. This said this, many disregard the importance of nutrition in this sport, and also how much they could benefit from a good planning, saving them shots.

A round of golf is played on 18 holes and lasts from 4 to 5 hours, while the average course is about 7 Km. A golfer may walk 9-10 Km to complete an 18-holes round. During the week professional golfers may stay up to 8 hours a day on a court, while training on specific abilities and strokes or practicing. Physical training, including strength exercises, aerobic conditioning, flexibility, are usually part of professional golfers' training sessions, helping them to strengthen specific muscles involved in the game, to improve their resistance and to reduce injury risks. Pros undergo such a training at least 3 times a week, for minimum 3 hours. Gold tournaments develop in rounds of 18 holes within 4 consecutive days, and, during a season, a pro may take part up to 25 tournaments, this being 100 rounds in 100 days of competitions a year (Fig.1).

RANK	PGA TOUR	EVENTI	ROUNDS	EUROPEAN TOUR	EVENTI	ROUNDS
1	Rory McIlroy	19	76	RAHM, Jon	13	52
2	Brooks Koepka	21	84	FLEETWOOD, Tommy	18	72
4	Justin Thomas	20	80	WIESBERGER, Bernd	30	120
3	Jon Rahm	20	80	LOWRY, Shane	15	60
6	Xander Schauffele	21	84	FITZPATRICK, Matthew	20	80
5	Rickie Fowler	20	80	MCILROY, Rory	13	72
7	Adam Scott	18	72	WALLACE, Matt	27	108
8	Justin Rose	17	68	OOSTHUIZEN, Louis	14	48
9	Gary Woodland	24	96	HATTON, Tyrrell	18	72
10	Matt Kuchar	22	88	VAN ROOYEN, Erik	29	116
11	Webb Simpson	21	84	MACINTYRE, Robert	31	124
12	Jason Day	21	84	KINHULT, Marcus	25	100
13	Patrick Cantlay	21	84	PEREZ, Victor	26	104
14	Paul Casey	22	88	KITAYAMA, Kurt	31	124
15	Adam Hadwin	24	96	WILLETT, Danny	14	48
16	Scott Piercy	24	96	HEBERT, Benjamin	27	108
17	Sungjae Im	35	140	SCHWAB, Matthias	29	116
18	Hideki Matsuyama	24	96	BEZUIDENHOUT, Christiaan	28	112
19	Bry. DeChambeau	21	84	LORENZO-VERA, Mike	22	88
20	Sam Ryder	23	92	CAMPILLO, Jorge	28	112

Fig. 1 – rounds playes in 2019 by the top 10 PGA Tour and European Tour pros

(from www.europeantour.com and www.pgatour.com)

The leading tournaments of the European Tour go from January to November ; this means that pros are touring the world for most of the year. Their schedules are extremely tight : while the competition is facing its final moments on a given Sunday, most of the players go from changing rooms to airports, after the following tournament. The schedule can be relentless for pros, and all these flights, jet-lags, international food increase the risk of illnesses both for them and for their caddies. Nutritional support should therefore be periodized focusing on the requirements of their daily training and of overall nutritional scopes. The purpose of nutrition during training sessions will be to promote the adjustments during the training, while the focus of nutrition during competitions will be to give the best performance during the tournament.

To sum up, professional golfers are real athletes, who undergo a substantial physical and mental workload for a great part of the year. This workload needs to be scheduled to avoid having a performance decrease during the final part of the Tour. A balanced nutritional programme should be put in place at the very beginning of the professional career, after an extensive evaluation of the energetic and nutritional status of the athlete.

1

The energy expenditure of a golf player

Playing golf involves long bouts of walking, which are marked by an energy expenditure linked to the walking speed, the distance and the ascents and descents of the court (*Stauch M, Liu Y, Giesler M. et al, 1999*). These walking sessions are interchanged with the swinging sessions, which can have different technical features and whose energy expenditure may be hard to quantify, due to the extreme short duration of the technical gesture. (Fig.2)

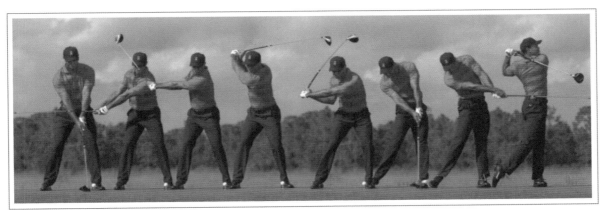

Fig.2: the technical gesture of the World's greatest player of all times: Tiger Wood's swing (from Golf Digest).

According to the American College of Sports Medicine (ACSM) guidelines to classify the intensity of physical activity (*ACSM's guidelines for exercise testing, 2009; Ainsworth, B., Haskell, W.L et al., 2000*), golf goes from low to vigorous intensity (3-6 METS) (*Luscombe J,Murray AD et al., 2017*).

The average heart rate during the game goes from 48,5% to 67,4% of HR max (Fig. 3). The average round is 227 minutes and golfers can walk around 9,000 metres. They spend most of the time with a moderate-intensity physical activity : 82 minutes with 50-74% of maximum heart rate (*Luscombe J,Murray AD et al., 2017*). There is, nevertheless, a large gap between medium and maximum heart rate. This is linked to temporary physical needs linked both to the athlete's body and to golf itself.

Studies carried out on non-professional golfers show that an average non-professional player burns appr. 2,500 calories during a 18-hole golf game (*Burkett LN, von Heijne-Fisher U et al., 2017; Zunzer SC, von Duvillard SP et al., 2013*).

	TIME (min)	AVERAGE FC (bpm)	%FC MAX	Kcal
AVERAGE	227	105-128	48,5-67,4	2500
CASE	287	118	61.7	2810

Fig. 3: Energy expenditure for a 18-hole round in the average data of literature (AVERAGE) and our sample case (CASE)

As you know, the Total Daily Energy Expenditure (TDEE) is a calculation of your Resting Energy Expenditure (REE) plus your Activity Energy Expenditure (AEE):

TDEE = REE + AEE

The Resting Energy Expenditure (REE) represents the amount of energy needed by an organism at rest, both for its maintenance and for digestive processes, that is the sum of Basal Metabolic Rate (BMR) and the energy you need to digest food (Thermic Effect of Food – TEF):

REE = BMR + TEF

The Basal Metabolic Rate (BMR) Calculator, as previously explained, estimates the amount of energy needed to maintain the basal metabolic activities, such as body temperature and vital organs maintenance (which include brain, kidneys, heart and lungs). Basal metabolic values are significantly influenced by, among others, body composition, sex, body temperature, age, energy restriction, genetics and endocrine system. It can be measured with indirect calorimetry, which defines Resting Energy Expenditure (REE) thanks to the measurement of oxygen consuption (VO2) and carbon dioxyde production (VCO2) (*Haugen HA, Chan LN et al., 2007*) or simply using equations which give satisfactory esteems (*Jagim AR, Camic CL et al., 2018*).

The Activity Energy Expenditure (AEE) is the only element of the energy expenditure we can accurately control and it represents 20-40% of the Total Daily Energy Expenditure (TDEE) related to the Physical Activity Level (PAL). We need to consider a PAL value starting from 2,4 on for a professional athlete (*Hills PA , Mokhtar N. et al., 2014*).

In general, we can classify physical activities on the basis of their theoretical energy expenditure, defining it in MET, as displayed by literature (*Ainsworth BE, Haskell WL, et al., 1993*). Activities with an energy expenditure of 1,5 MET are considered light by Ainsworth and coll., while those with an expenditure of 4 and 6 MET are considered moderate and intense.

Ultimately, the player's daily calorie requirement depends on genetic inheritance, age, weight, body composition, daily training and on training schedule

1.1 The sample case

Our case study is a professional athlete of the pro European Tour. It is a 24 year-old male, 80 Kg body weight, with a very active lifestyle, a medium-high intense training of about 14 hours a week (golf practice) and about 3 hours a week of work out.

We start by calculating his BMR, using Harris Benedict (*Roza AM, Shizgal HM, 1984*) formula, which gives us a value of 1,970 Kcal. Multiplying the BMR value with the physical activity level (PAL), we have an estimation of his daily energy expenditure :
In this particular case we multiply the BMR by 2.2 (medium-high activity for a professional athlete), thus obtaining 4,351 Kcal :

BMR * 2,2 = 1970 * 2 = 4351 Kcal

We calculated the energy expenditure during a pro competition, monitoring 12 rounds (18 holes) during 3 consecutive competitions (4 rounds per competition). The average duration of each round was 287 minutes (287.3 ± 23.6). The average heart rate, tested with continuous monitoring system WHOOP™ (Fig.4 e 5), was 118 bpm (118.6 ± 5.6), that's to say 61.7% of maximal HR. The average calorie expenditure obtained using Keytel's formula (*Keytel LR, Goedecke JH , 2005*) was 587 Kcal/h, that is 2,810 Kcal per round. Using the above energy expenditure elements, we can say that the Total Energy Expenditure value for a competition day is 4,713 Kcal :

REE + AEE = 1903 + 2810 = 4713 Kcal

Ultimately, a competition day requires 4,713 Kcal on average, compared to a regular training day of 4,351 Kcal, with 362 Kcal more. It is therefore essential for the athlete to satisfy his caloric needs during both training sessions and competitions, in order to be able to improve performances and to keep a good health condition. The lack of assumption of the right quantities of energy can lead to a loss of muscle mass, performance decrease, recovery complications and higher fatigue risk, injuries and illnesses (Burke, L.M., Close, G.L *et al., 2018*).

Once we have defined the total energy expenditure during a competition day or a typical training day, we can set up an appropriate dietary schedule. Individual nutritional requirements will be determined according to training loads, the athlete's specific needs, training goals and body composition goals.

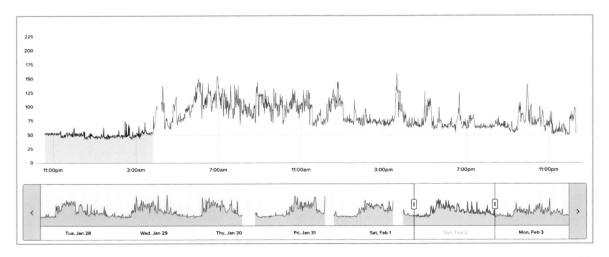

Fig.4 Heart rate continuous monitoring system with WHOOP™ (Whoop, Boston, Massachusetts, USA)

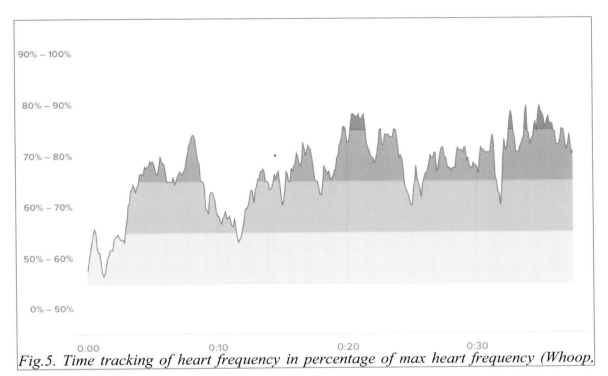

Fig.5. Time tracking of heart frequency in percentage of max heart frequency (Whoop, Boston, Massachusetts, USA).

2

Evaluation of the nutritional status and of the body composition

The evaluation of the physical and nutritional status of a golf player includes a general medical examination, along with some specific blood chemistry tests, body composition and eating habits investigation.

The player's anamnesis involves information about the player's and his family's pre-existing conditions, as well as his physiological status. The family history is helpful, when it comes to the investigation of illnesses in more than one member of the family, and it guides in the research of hereditary diseases or food intolerances. As far as the invidual is concerned, you need to examine not only past injuries or digestive conditions, but also if these may interfere with the training. The investigation of the athletic background must indentify the intensity and duration of the training in a typical week and the competitive commitment during the year.

The following step is the study of eating habits, which is key to get information about the causes of a potential nutritional disease (*Bean A, 2013*).

This should be done by esteeming the amount of nutrients the athlete ingests. Because a pro golf player travels in different countries with various nutrients availabilies, we should give up making a detailed calculation of each single nutrient assumption and be content with an approximation. You can obtain it by asking information on the type of food, the number of meals, and the quantity of food ingested. You can obtain these data with sufficient reliability thanks to a journal of the previous 24 hours and a questionnaire on consumption frequency (All. 1).

Ultimately, you can give more specific recommendations on the athlete's nutritional needs once you know the intensity and the time committed to his athletic activity, his physiological factors, and his eating habits.

Biochemical and haematological tests are key in evaluating the golfer's nutritional status. Specimen are usually obtained from blood, urine and faeces.

These tests help you figure out the concentration of nutrients (glucose, lipids, albumin, minerals, vitamins, etc), metabolites (urea, creatinine, etc), enzymes involved in several pathways of metabolism, some indirect indicators connected to nutrients utilizations (haemoglobin and haematocrit, transferrin), but also possible situations of immunodeficiency (leukocyte, etc).

We recommend these blood and urinary tests to be part of a first diagnosis: complete blood count and differential, fasting blood glucose, serum creatinine and azotemia, blood electrolytes, AST, ALT, total cholesterol, LDL, HDL, triglyceride, sideremia, transferrin, ferritin, TSH, Vit D, Vit B12.

A periodic check of these exams and their correct interpretation, which integrate the clinical history and the nutritional evaluation, help identify and fix deficiencies which may influence the general health status and the athletic performance. An in-depth analysis on intestinal microbiota should be done with a specific fecal examination, which gives precise information on the player's intestinal flora, which, as we will see, is very important for the athlete.

The following step to correctly assess the athlete's condition is the analysis of the golfer's body composition through Body Impedance Analysis. Body Impedance Analysis is a method based on the behaviour of the human body's biological structures when a weak electric current flows through it (*Moon JR., 2013*). Measuring the two elements of human body's impedance (resistance and reactance) during the current flow, BIA allows us to calculate : Total Body Water (TBW), IntraCellular Water (ICW), ExtraCellular Water (ECW), Fat Mass (FM) and Fat-Free Mass (FFM), subdivided in ExtraCellular Mass (ECM) and Body Sell Mass (BCM), and Muscolar Mass (MM) (Fig.6).

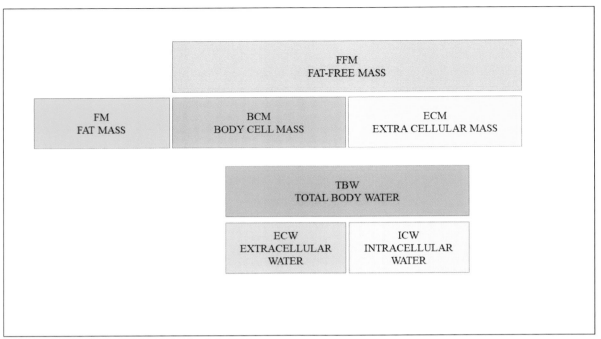

Fig.6 Parameters measured with BIA.

It's essential to monitor the player's body composition throughout time, both during training session and immediately before a round. This enables you to check if any variations are linked to the variation of Active Cellular Mass or Fat Mass, loss or gain of water, and allows you to fine-tune training programmes, adapt diet and keep the ideal hydration to improve the performance.

As far as a golf player is concerned, it is important to check BCM and MM and the way they change during training sessions, to avoid decreases that may occur during too intense or prolongued trainings, or due to inappropriate diet (Fig. 5). A high BCM (appr. 50% of FFM) is seen as a target, if you want to improve the player's physical conditions and athletic performances.

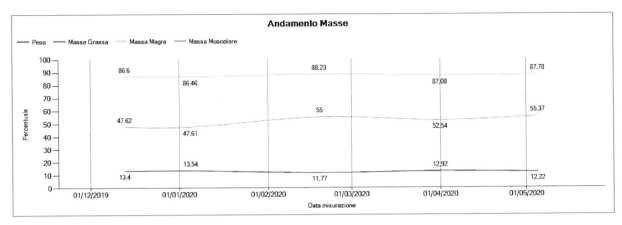

Fig. 7: Bio-electrical impedance time develompment of the values of FM, FFM and MM (Gedip, Eupraxia srl, Reggio Emilia, Italy).

Bio-electrical impedance is extremely useful to assess the state of hydration in the athlete. A slight dehydration can lead to significant decreases in the sports performance (*Cheuvront SN, Kenefick RW, 2014*). Experiencing an ideal extracellular hydration before a round or a training session results in lower risks of muscolar traumatic events (ECW about 45% of TBW) and you can also benefit from a faster recover of your physical conditions after the training. If you know these data and their trend, you can act ahead of time to keep an optimal hydration state (ECW 40-50% of TBW) without jeopardizing the performance (Fig. 7 e 8)

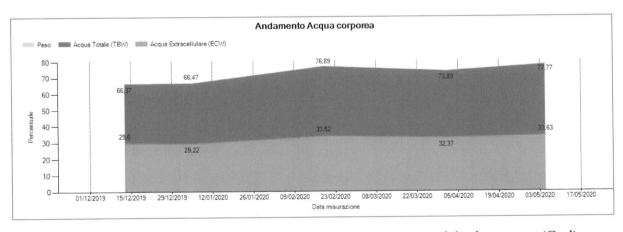

Fig. 8: Bio-electrical impedance analysis time development of body water (Gedip, Eupraxia srl, Reggio Emilia, Italy)

3

Macronutrients

We already have guidelines on the amount of nutrients an athlete should consume, if he wants to optimize his performance (*Thomas DT, Erdman KA, 2016; Vitale K, Getzin A, 2019*).

Adapting this information to the specific needs of every golf player is fundamental if we want to develop a customized nutritional programme.

A professional golf player's diet should therefore include this amount of macronutrients: 7-12 grams of carbs per Kg body weight, 1.2-1.7 grams of proteins per Kg of body weight and approximately 20-30% of overall intake of fats. This satisfies all nutritional needs, both if you are trying to gain or lose body weight, as well as maintaining your body weight, being the total intake of calories the only variation.

3.1 Carbohydrates

Carbohydrates are classified in two different categories, depending on their chemical structure : simple (sugars) and complex (starch, fibres). Simple carbs include glucose, saccarose, galactose, lactose. Among complex carbs (a compound of many molecules, mainly glucose, stuck together) we have starches, amylose, amylopectine, fibres. We also have a middle ground: glucose polymers and maltodextrines (common in sports drink), which are composed by 3-10 glucose molecules. We use the glycemic index to study the effects of all carbs on levels of glucose in the blood (blood glucose), that is to measure how fast a food is digested and converted into glucose. We have a table of food items (Fig. 9) with correlated values from 0 to 100, depending on their effect on blood glucose (the higher the value, the faster the rise in blood sugar) (*Atkinson FS, Foster-Powell K, et al., 2008*).

LOW GI	Apples peaches, legumes, fructose, ice-creams, milk, yoghurt.
MODERATE GI	spaghetti and pasta in general, dry biscuits, grapes, oranges.
HIGH GI	Glucose, saccharose (white sugar) and simple sugars including maltodextrines, honey, bananas, white wheat bread, cornflakes, rice.

Fig.9: Glycemic index of most common food items (reworked by Bean A. The complete guide to sport nutrition. 2013, Bloomsbury Publishing, London)

The biggest disadvantage of the glycemic index is that it does not take the portion sizes of foods into consideration; we should therefore use the Glycemic Load to obtain a more accurate value of the rise in sugar blood:

GI = (glycemic index * grams of carbs/100).

All athletes, including golf players, produce less insulin when consuming high GI foods, so glycemic index should be used only to have a general idea about the impact of a specific food item on the body (*Bean A., 2013*).

Glucose is stocked in the liver and muscles. Storages of glycogen are limited and can fuel the body only for some hours during a medium-high aerobic training such as golf (*Tarnopolsky MA, Gibala M, et al., 2005*). It is important to underline that, when glycogen levels decrease, the intensity and the perfomance decrease as well. The simplest guideline for a gold player to maximise gycogen levels is to eat appropriate quantities of carbs, depending on the training intensity and volume. Carbs recommended daily consumptions are usually between 5-12 g/kg/day. The top end (8-10g/kg/day) is meant for athletes with a moderate-high intensity training ($\geq$ 70% VO2max) for more than 12 hours a week (*Howarth KR, Moreau NA, 2009*).

A golf player needs to be sure that his glycogen supplies are high before the training, if he wants to achieve his best performance. When scheduling the diet, you should calculate the carbs needs not only on body weight, but also on the training volume, because the storage capacity is proportional to muscle mass and body weight (*Burke L., 2007*); so the heavier the body muscle, the higher the storage capacity of glycogen, the higher the training load, the higher the request for carbs (Fig.10). In this way you can calculate the need for carbs, regardless of the daily intake of calories.

Work load	Need of carbs
Low intensity	3-5 grams per kilo
Medium intensity	5-7 grams per kilo
Medium-high intensity (max 3 hours/day)	7-12 grams per kilo
High intensity (over 4 hours/day)	10-12 grams per kilo

Fig. 10 Daily intake of carbs (taken from Burke L. Pratical Sports Nutrition, Human Kinetics, Champaign, IL, 2007)

3.2 Proteins

Proteins give the units that build all tissues thanks to their constituent amino acids. Athletes use food proteins to repair and rebuild their skeletal muscle and their connecting tissues after training sessions or competitions. Proteins also help maintain fluid balance, transport nutrients and oxygen, and regulate blood clotting.

They are built up of amino acids that join together, in many different ways. There are 12 non essential amino acids, which can be formed by our body, and 8 essential ones, which come from the food we eat. Protein sources containing higher levels of essential amino acids are considered high level proteins. Atheles have several protein sources, each one having pros and cons. Along with essential amino acids, fats, calories, micronutrients and various bioactive peptides, all contribute to the quality of a protein.

Professional athletes need a bigger amount of proteins compared to the average population, and this helps them compensate the increase of proteic degradation during physical exercise and repair the muscle tissue after the training (*Phillips SM, 2004*).

The recommended amount of proteins for endurance athletes is 1,2-2.0 grams per kilo per day (*Phillips SM, 2014*). In order to estimate the daily amount of proteins, you need to carefully size up different elements linked to training programme, age, body composition, training status, as well as the total energy supply of the diet, especially for those athletes, who want to loose fat weight and limit calories to achieve this goal (*Jäger et al., 2017*). You should not forget that protein degradation also takes place when the supply of glycogen is limited or in case of a diet with a reduced carbohydrate level. Golf players should satisfy their protein need with a well balanced diet, which provides the right amount of calories. Most athletes follow diets, which give them an intake of protein, higher than the recommended value, even without protein supplements (*Jäger et al., 2017*). Vegetarian athletes can benefit from low-fat dairy and vegetable sources rich in proteins to satisfy their needs.

3.3 **Fats**

Fats and oils in food are composed by triglycerides generated by the combination of one molecule of glycerol with three fatty acids. Depending on their chemical structure, fatty acids can be divided in saturated, monounsaturated and polyunsaturated; they are broken down to produce energy (Fig.11). Dietary fats contain over twice the energy (9 kcal/gram) of carbs (4 kcal/gram). A diet with 20-30% of energy coming from fat is usually recommended (*Rodriguez NR, Di Marco NM, 2009*). Even though there have been attempts to change the proportion of fat in diets, there seems to be no reason to move away from the adviced 30%, mainly for health reasons.

SATURATED	Solid at room temperature	Butter, lard, cheese	10%
MONOUNSATURATED	Liquid at room temperature, but they can solidify at low temperature	Olive oil, peanut oil, almond oil, seeds oil	12%
POLYUNSATURATED	Liquid both at room and at low temperature	Vegetable oils, fish oil, oily fish	10%

Fig. 11: Fatty acids and their percentage in the diet.

As far as athletes are concerned, you should be careful about polyunsaturates in Omega-3, because they might influence not only the physical activity and the metabolic response of the skeletal muscle, but also the functional response to a training period. Health and performance improvement can also benefit from their potential anti-inflammatory and antioxidant activity (*Gammone MA, Riccioni G et al, 2018*). Golf players experience long periods of physiological stress, associated with transient inflammations, oxidative stress and perturbations of immune responses, as their physical exercise activates multiple molecular and biochemical pathways, which involve the immune system and are susceptible to nutrition (*Philpott JD, Witard OC, 2019*).

Nutritional support can therefore partially mitigate the changes linked to exercise. The most effective nutritional countermeasures for athletes include the consumption of Omega-3 and antioxidants, such as vitamins, carotenoids, polyphenols, probiotics. Omega-3 supplements seem to be the most useful ones, not only for athletes but also for the general population.

3.4 The sample case

Going back to our golf athlete, once we calculate the average needs for a training day and for a competition day, we can determine the nutrient intakes with the following guidelines : 8 gr/Kg of carbs, 1.8 gr/Kg of proteins and 1.6 gr/Kg of fats. This leads us to a balanced diet with 60% of the caloric intake coming from carbs, 13% from proteins and 27% from fats, that is 651.6 grams of carbs, 141.1 grams of proteins and 130.3 grams of fats.

The next step is to distribute them during the whole day, and we suggest 5 meals (breakfast, snack, lunch, snack, dinner), with the following caloric distribution : 25-5-40-5-25. This gives us the opportunity to set up a customized diet.

4

Micronutrients

Vitamins and minerals are essential for many metabolic processes, as they are involved in chemical reactions linked to carbs utilization, fat and protein metabolism (*Burke L, Heeley P, 2000*). They need to be included in the diet, as they are not produced by the human body. As far as athletes are concerned, their need has always been a matter of debate. Some experts state that athletes need more vitamins and minerals compared to sedentary population, while others claim they don't (*American College of Sports Medicine, 2000*). It is true that most athletes eat more than sedentary people, thus increasing both substances. Intensity, duration and frequency of training, connected with total energy and nutrients consumption certainly influence the higher or lower need of micronutrients (*Burke L, Heeley P, 2000; Thomas DT, Erdman KA, et al, 2016*). Being on a balanced diet is not always easy for a golf player, who travels both frequently and abroad, where he may find unfamiliar food. It is therefore possible that he does not always eat all the vitamins and minerals he needs, especially if his intake of fruit, vegetables and dairy products is low. We need to highlight that both scarse reserves and insufficient intakes of micronutrients may lead to negative effects on the performance. On the other hand vitamin and mineral supplements in quantities exceeding the needs have no benefit on it either (*Thomas DT, Erdman KA, et al, 2016*). There might be players whose needs of micronutrients are higher, due to an excessive drop, for instance with sweat and urines. You might take a supplement into consideration in such cases. Only players with low quantitites of specific micronutrients can, in the end, benefit from their supplementation, in terms of nutritional status and athletic performance. This is even more true for athletes, who are on low-calorie diets, because they need to supplement them with acceptable intakes of iron, calcium, magnesium, zinc and vitamin B12 (*Kondo S, Tanisawa K, et al., 2019*).

5

Nutrition for golf

We need to carefully consider the athletic activity of a professional golf player on a nutritional point of view, because of the varied use of muscle masses (walking and swinging) and the high mental commitment (putting).

There are no such things as magic food or specific diets that can improve the golfer's athletic performance. Only a healthy and adequate nutrition can contribute to a more efficient body, enabling it to face trainings and competitions appropriately, without any risk. Some golf players believe that sports nutrition rules do not apply to them, that they can manage a competition with minimum or zero preparatory dietary adjustment, but in fact quite the opposite is true. Due to the fact that golf players play a round a day for many days in a row, it is impossible to achieve good results without the right amounts of nutrients. A top-level performance requires a well-structured diet, both in the daily training and in a competition scenario.

A professional competition lasts a week: the first three days (Monday, Tuesday and Wednesday) are focused on the practical and mental approach and on the study of the court, whereas the other four days (Thursday, Friday, Saturday and Sunday) to the competition itself, made of 4 consecutive rounds, each of 18 holes (Fig.12).

The total amount of carbs in the body (muscle and hepatyc glycogen) is limited, and it is certainly not enough if we compare it to such an intense and on-going activity. You need to think that a competition day requires a good warm-up session, which can last 60 minutes, a 4-5 hour tour, where you can walk up to 7 Km and some training after the round. This takes place every single day for many days in a row during the Tour. Having the right amount of carbs gives you the energy you need to be able to play and to perform well at the end of the round (the last holes), and, moreover, towards the end of the tournament (the weekend).

We need to consider a typical week, but we should not forget that golf competitions take place one after the other, week after week, often including long, even intercontinental, plane trips. This specific situation has to be taken into account, as these transfers can influence physical conditions, especially towards the end of the Tour, which is not only the most challenging time, but also the one where the player has to give his best, both on the athletic and the mental point of view. It is therefore essential to plan the diet for the whole season, differentiating the first part, the second part and the final part, setting clear goals in terms of weight and body composition.

As far as the diet of the golf player is concerned, we need to identify his training or daily diet and his competition diet. The competition diet has three moments: the pre-competition, the competition, the post competition.

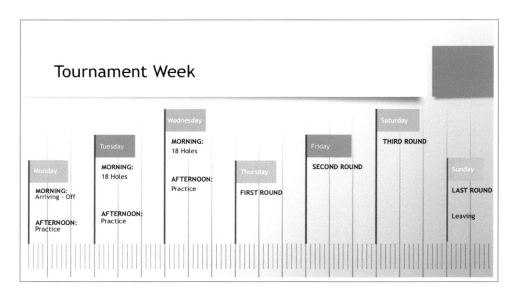

Fig. 12: A typical "schedule" of a professional golf round

5.1 The training session

The distinctive feature of the diet at this stage is the increase of the energy need connected to the increase of the energy consumption linked to the athletic activity.

The golf player, who pursuits his sport with commitment and consistency, must rely on a feed ration distribution during the day, which might be really consistent, so that it does not interfere with the training sessions.

The diet, appreciated and easy to digest, should be mainly composed by carbs (55-60% of the daily total energy). Most of these (80%) should be complex carbs, such as those you can find in cereals (pasta, bread, biscuits, rusks, rice, corn, etc.) and in tubers (potatoes). The other 20% of the carb rate is made by simple sugars (white sugar, honey, jams, sweets, fruit, etc.). Carbs set up the primary energy substrate for exercising muscles, and they are therefore suitable for rapid and intense sporting gestures (swing), and for lasting ones (walking).

A golf player's average protein need is 1.2-1.8 grams per kg bodyweight, especially when the activity is not only a lasting one, but also daily and with a high muscle effort (gym activity and practice) (*Kondo S, Tanisawa K, 2019*).

Proteins count for 12-15% of the total calories in a golfer's daily ration, and they should come both from vegetables like legumes, such as chickpeas, beans, peas, etc., and cereals, such as pasta, rice, etc., and from food of animal origin (milk and dairy products, meat, fish, eggs, etc.), with a slight predominance of better iron sources (haem-iron), much better absorbed and bio-available for the human body.

Fats, together with carbs, are a fundamental energy source when it comes to a lasting physical activity (over 20-30 minutes of non-stop muscle activity) of medium-high intensity (equal to or higher than 70% of the VO2 max). According to the circumstances, they should count for a flexible percentage, between 25% and 30% of the daily total energy, eaten both as fats contained in food, and as seasonings. As far as the last ones are concerned, those from vegetables should be preferred, especially virgin olive oil and extra virgin olive oil, more easily digestible and rich in substances with an antioxidant action. (*Ørtenblad N, Westerblad H, 2013*).

The golfer diet, preferably inspired by the Mediterranean Diet, should therefore be composed by different types of food, rich in fruit and vegetables, both raw or cooked, to guarantee an adequate supply of water, mineral salts, vitamins, antioxidants and dietary fibers.

5.2 The pre-competition session

We define the pre-competition period as the one forerunning by three-four hours the start from hole 1 tee. We need from three to four hours to digest a meal, and this means that you need to eat in this time interval before the start, so that the digestion is over and both the glycemic peak and the insuline response are back to normal. High insulin levels due to carbs and proteins intake, may, on the other hand, lead to adverse effects on the athletic performance, determined by reflex hypoglycemia (*Zouhal H, Jacob C, Delamarche P, et al 2008*).

A good pre-competition meal should include food rich in carbs, to maximise glycogen stores, low contents of fats and fibers, to facilitate the gastric emptying and minimise the gastrointestinal disorders, a moderate amount of proteins, and, most of all, must be familiar and well tolerated, as a result of previous tests. The suggested amount of carbs is between 1-4 grams per kilogram body weight (*Bean A., 2013*), but 2,5 mg/kg can be used in most cases (*Thomas DT, Erdman KA, 2016*).

Most of the carbohydrate intake must come from generous rations of complex ones, the so-called starches. Among these we should mention pasta, especially durum wheat pasta, rice, potatoes, bread and other bakery products (dry biscuits, saltines, breadsticks, rusks, etc), as well as cereals (corn, barley, spelt, etc) and legumes, even though you should be careful to avoid possible digestive discomforts (swelliness, flatulence, rapid intestinal emptying) caused by incomplete digestion of the dietary fiber highly contained in these products. Simple sugars will, therefore, be a rather low percentage (20%) of the total carboydrate amount, but undoubtely generous, if you compare it to the total daily calory intake of the feed ration.

It is nonetheless very difficult to estimate the amount of food a golf player needs before a tournament, as tolerances vary considerably from person to person. Some players like to eat a balanced meal made of good carbs, but also fats and good proteins, such as eggs, in order not to fell hungry in the last session of the round. Golfers' rounds can last even more than 5 hours, so it is important to have a sufficiently nourishing meal, in order to maintain constant blood sugar and energy levels, and to avoid fatigue.

Meal time depends on tee time. As tee time changes, golf players must develop a nutritional plan, which can adapt to the different timings. Every athlete is different, but their meals should basically include carbs and liquids for hydration. A small quantity of proteins is also good, as it helps avoid hunger during a possibly long round. Those, who might be nervous or hungry before competing, can have a liquid supply of proteins and carbs, like a fruit smoothie.

Should the round start early in the morning, consider the following : hepatic glycogen, which is mainly used to keep blood sugar levels normal, is labile and it can drain the night before the competition. Beginning to exercise early in the morning, with a low blood sugar level might lead to premature fatigue (*Ørtenblad N, Westerblad H, et al, 2013*),

so eating before a competition taking place in the first hours of the day is mandatory. If you cannot wake up 4 hours before leaving, then you had better eat a small snack 30-90 minutes before beginning the activity, keeping in mind to eat the right quantity of carbs the evening before, to maximise glycogen supplies.

Players may also have another small snack 1 hour before the tee time. This snack is usually a light one and it is full of carbs, but low in fats and fibers, which makes it easy to digest. This snack serves to overcome hypoglycemia and an increase of glycogenolysis in muscles in the first 30-60 minutes of the competition, as well as to decrease the psychic stress before the competition and to oppose the glucose lowering effect of adrenaline, which happens in such situations. This helps keeping constant and excellent blood sugar levels (*Coggan AR, Coyle EF, 2011).*

Glucose and sucrose, a disaccharide that is formed by glucose and fructose, have long been banned from athletes' pre-competition meals, because of the above-mentioned adverse effects on glucose and fat metabolism. These are linked to hyperinsulinaemia that follows their ingestion (*Murray B, Rosenbloom, 2018).*

Energy drinks based on maltodextrin (glucose polymers) could be very useful in this situation, specifically for their chemical and nutritional properties. Probably, they are today's best nutritional choice when it comes to waiting meals to be taken in the hours prior the physical exercise, no matter the metabolic workload. A possible waiting meal is a 4-6% isotonic solution of maltodextrin, to contain dehydration, which starts even before the athletic effort itself.

5.3 **The competition session**

We want all nutritional levels to be stable during a competition. The lenght of golf rounds requires athletes to eat and drink during the competition, to be able to face dehydration and hunger, to facilitate the energy recharge of muscles, thus avoiding an exhaustion of muscle glycogen. We have already said that muscles mainly rely on carbs as fuel source during medium-high intensity exercise (*Murray B, Rosenbloom,2018; Burke L*, 2011). Professional golf is played with 60-65% of VO2max, and must therefore be considered a medium-high intensity sport. Many researches have studied the speed needed by the body to use carbs during the training and, even though many aspects slightly influence this rate, we generally agree on the way the body can metabolize 1 single gram of carbs per minute (*Coyle EF, 1998*). A lower intake might not give enough energy to sustain an ideal work rate in muscles. On the other hand, a considerable amount can lead to gastrointestinal discomfort, which can put the athletic performance at risk. One example is the intake of sugary drinks, whose aim is to give enough carbs to maintain the blood sugar and the carbohydrate oxidation with neither gastrointestinal alterations nor fluid uptake gap. The performance is usually better with a carbs intake of 30-60 g/hour (*Burke L*, 2011; *Coyle EF, 1998*).

Solid food needs to be eaten regularly and must be divided in small portions, not heavier than 50 grams. It must mainly contain complex carbs with very low intake of simple sugars, as these are usually highly contained in drinks. Proteins and fats (milk, low-fat fresh cheese, eggs) can be included, even though in very small quantities, to make portions more palatable and easier to chew.

Liquid portions are a better and more convenient option, especially with an addition of sugars and minerals, such as glucose, saccharose, or, even better, maltodextrin (*Hao, L.; Chen, Q , et al., 2014*) while fructose is not recommended, due to the digestive disorders mentoned before.

It is important to highlight that there is no difference between the intake of sugary drinks and of solid portions containing carbs, as far as their effect on performance or the strain holdup is concerned.

The average duration of a round is 287 minutes, that is to say 16 minutes per hole. It is therefore fundamental to have a break every 4 holes, eating the already recommended 30 grams of carbs, to be able to boost energy levels and stay focused. It is also very important to engage the caddy, making him part of the nutritional plan, so that he can remind the player to eat regularly (ex. hole 4, 8, 12, 16).

The frequency of carbs intake can be obtained without compromising the liquid one, drinking 600/1200 ml of drinking solution containing from 4% to 8% of carbs per 100 ml. We have already said that carbs can be sugars (glucose or saccharose) or amids (maltodextrin) *(Hao, L.; Chen, Q , et al., 2014)*. A basic requirement of hydrosaline supplements must be their hypotonicity or isotonocity (250-300 mOsm) compared to plasma values, to avoid the attraction of water in the digestive system, resulting in a general dehydration, gastric emptying and intestinal absorption. The inclusion of simple carbs is driven by the proven effectiveness of how small amounts of sugars can improve hydro-salt absorption. This is the reason why you can therefore use monosaccharides up to 5% max and disaccharides and higher polymers up to 10%, but also why you should not exceed the limits of osmolarity *(Bean A., 2013)*.

5.4 **The post competition session**

Once the competition is over you need to replenish both water and saline losses caused by sweating, and restock the sugar (muscle and hepatic glycogen) needed to sustain the muscle energetic effort. Nutrition aimed at recovering the strength is essential for a professional golf player, who is engaged in four rounds in a row in four days.

It is better to choose hydro-mineral supplements added with sugars (maltodextrine, glucose, saccharose) powdered if possible, to be able to measure the quantity of sugar according to single needs.

The consumption of liquids straight after the training can be quantified according to the change of weight before and after the physical activity, adding another 50% of the weight change, to face the amount of water which will be lost with urines: for instance, if a player looses 1 kg during the competition, he will have to drink 1 + ½ liter.

You usually need about 20 hours to restore muscle glycogen supplies almost completely, but you will need more time if the food intake of carbs is not sufficient (*Burke L*, 2011*)*.

The intake of 1 gram of glucose per kg of body weight straight after activity within the first two hours, increases the glycogen synthesis at a higher speed, compared to what would happen if it started after two hours (*Burke L*, 2011*)*. It is therefore fundamental to persuade players to eat carbs as soon as possible after the competition, avoiding going to the driving range, but dedicating the first two hours to nutritional restoration.

What we have just stated confirms the recommendation to eat snacks and/or heavily sweetened supplements (1-1,5 gr per kg of body weight) as quickly as possible after a muscle strain. The intake of about 0.7-1.5 gr of glucose per kg of body weight short after the activity, done every 2 hours for the first 6 hours, results in a total intake of 600 gr of carbs (appr. 10 gr/kg of body weight) during the 24 hours following activity, giving the player the maximum speed of resynthesis of muscle glycogen.

Athletes should go for food with a higher glycemic index during the recovery phase (simple sugar), whereas, as already seen, they should choose those with a lower glycemic index when eating before the activity.

Recovery meals and snacks should also include a lot of liquids and elettrolites, to replace perspiration, and some proteins, to « repair » muscles, along with carbs. Compared to carbs only, a blend of carbs and proteins has proven to be better in facilitating the reintegration of glycogen supplies. Blends stimulate a higher release of insulin, which speeds up the muscle cells uptake of glucose and amino acids from blood. They not only boost protein and glycogen synthesis, but they also reduce the increase of cortisol, which would rise after a competition, and which would stimulate the protein catabolism (Moore DR et al, *2009)*. The ideal post-competition meal or drink should contain 15-25 gr of proteins on average, to maximise the muscle restoration, and carbs, with a one-to-four ratio. We suggest to go for milk proteins, so that muscles can gain from a higher protein absorption. Milk is a perfect drink to promote recovery, both to reactivate glycogen supplies and to rehydrate (Wilkinson SB et al.., *2007)*.

6

Hydration

Playing conditions change significantly during the Tour season, but most tournaments take place during summer months and often in the hottest part of the day, thus highlighting the need for good habits as far as hydration is concerned. Players training or competing in hot-humid environments, in direct sunlight and with minimum airflow, have a high perspiration and risk dehydration (Maughan RJ, Shirreffs SM., *2010*).

Dehydration can lead to fatigue, reduced perfomance and reduced ability to concentrate for long periods (*McDermott BP, Anderson SA, et al, 2017).*

Golf involves competence and requires a high level of concentration for long hours. This means that it is fundamental that golf players drink enough to keep good hydration levels, both during competions and training. They should carry liquids in their golf bag and keep them cool to be more palatable.

Liquid needs increase with the heat, so golfers should check their sweating percentage to determine their needs for drinking. As already said, sports drinks or solutions of electrolytes replacements cans be useful when matched with long training rounds and competitions, as they contain fluids and electrolytes for hydrations and some carbs to satisfy the athletes' energy need.

The first thing to check is the quantity of fluids lost during the round, to be able to define both the quantity of the drink and the composition of salt supplements. The easiest way to determine lost fluids is to weigh the player before and after the activity. The variations of his body mass give a precise index of the water lost. It is imperative for a golf player to limit weigh loss to less than 1% of total body mass during the activity. Every player's weight and perspiration rate are different, so it is better to check the weight loss during the training to determine single specific fluids requirements (Cheuvront, S.N.; Kenefick, R.W , *2016; Sawka, M. N., Coyle E F.et al, 1999*). As a rule, weighing after micturition in the morning, with a measure of urine concentration, should give enough sensitivity (low false negative) to recognise any deviation in the balance of the body fluids (*Sawka, M. N., Coyle E F.et al, 1999*).

A practical aspect we should not overlook is that hydration affects the RR variability (HRV) ; dehydration especially reduces HRV, and this leads to a reduced parasympathetic activity, an increased sympathetic activity, or both. A sudden decrease of HRV during strenous rounds with high temperatures might show a dehydration we need to regulate (*McDermott, B.P.; Anderson, S.A et al., 2017*). Golf players usually drink less than they should during the activity, mostly because thirst is vague and it is influenced by many causes, including psychological ones and both nervous strain and mental effort distract from hydrating. Even if it is not easy to suggest how much a single person should drink, drinking 100 ml every 10 minutes of practice is nevertheless a good guideline. Players must drink according to an hydration plan before, during and after the competition, avoiding feeling thirsty. Researchers recommend that good hydration practices should include: 1) starting the exercise being euhydrated, 2) avoid excessive hypohydration during the activity and 3) replace losses after the last exercise and before the beginning of a new one (*Bergeron, M.F.; Bahr, R, et al., 2012; Racinais, S.; Alonso, J.M, et al., 2015; Sawka, M.N.; Coyle E., 2004*).

6.1 Pre-competition hydration

The aim of pre-hydration is starting a competition in good hydration having normal levels of plasmatic electrolydes. Players should be close to euhydration, if they drink sufficiently during their meals or if a prolonged recovery period has passed (8-12 h). A prehydration program will contribute to prevent any electrolydes deficiency before starting the physical activity. Otherwise, the performance will be affected by it.

You need to check both the hydration, the colour and the volume of urine, especially in hot and humid conditions. Thanks to the bioimpedance analysis it is easy to check the value of extra-cellular water ECW in previous days, bearing in mind that the ideal extra-cellular hydration before a competition or a training session amounts to 45%. In this condition the dehydration and the risk of muscle traumatic events are lower, and there will be a faster recovery speed after the training.

A fine-tuning of training and nutrition can lead the athlete to have perfect conditions. (Fig.13)

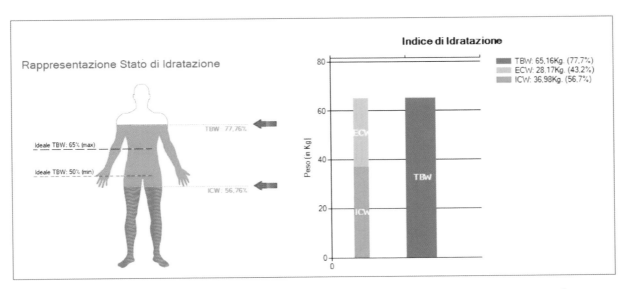

Fig. 13: graphic rapresentation of hydration measured with bioimpedance analysis (Software Gedip, Eupraxia srl, Reggio Emilia, Italy)

This is not always possible throughout the whole season, so you need to go for qualitative assessments. American College of Sports medicine – ACMS – recommends to drink 7 ml of liquids per kg of body weight at least 4 hours before the competition, to facilitate a good hydration and to give the body enough time to expell excess water. In case there is no diuresis within two hours or if urines are dark, you need to keep on drinking slowly (for example another ~ 3–5 mL/kg) approximately 2 hours before the event (*Castro-Sepúlveda M, Cerda-Kohler H, et al., 2015*).

Intaking water before a competition (pre-hydration) usually postpones dehydration, increases perspiration during the physical activity and delays the increase of body temperature. It is best to drink 500 ml of water at room temperature two hours before the beginning of the competition, especially with high temperatures. Pre-hydration does not cancel the need for a constant restoration of water during the physical effort. Athletes can drink other 250 ml 30 minutes before the competition, and other 250 ml 15 minutes before (Fig. 14)

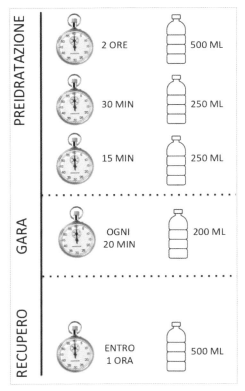

Fig. 14: Hydration planning for a golf tournament.

6.2 **Hydration during the competition**

Several studies showed that keeping an excellent performance is possible, if you re-integrate at least 80% of the loss in sweat during a competition (*Shirreffs, S. M., Maughan RJ, 1995*). The best approach is, as already said, weighting before and after the competition, and therefore drinking enough to reduce the loss of body weight within 1-2%.

During the training it is better to drink something fresh and palatable from a special container kept in the bag, which will be available to the caddie, who will remind the player to drink according to fixed times.

Most professional players drink 150-200 ml every 20 minutes. During the training, athletes prefer sugar drinks to water, so during a long golf round with no interruptions, having a sports drink with up to 8 gr of sugar per 100 ml instead of pure water, might positively influence the performance. In other words, you not only prevent dehydration, but also the premature decline of glycogen supplies and the sinking of blood-sugar, which are the three main causes of strain.

Carbs in sports drink not only give extra energy, but they also speed up water absorption : Hypotonic or isotonic solutions stimulate the absorption of water from the intestine and blood (concentration of sugar between 5 and 8 gr per 100 ml). More concentrated beverages (>8 gr per 100 ml), the ipotonic ones, help slow down the gastric emptying and therefore also the speed of liquids replenishing, and are not advisable.

Glucose polimers (matodextrin) are very useful and can be used in sports drinks instead of glucose and saccharose, as they help obtain a concentration up to 20 grams of carbohydrates per 100 ml, keeping the osmolarity of the solution low, thanks to the fact that the malodextrin molecule acts the same osmotic pressure of a glucose molecule, even though the quantity of glucose is higher.

6.3 **Post-competition hydration**

The water and sodium losses must be re-integrated after the competition, to keep the fluid balance normal. It is advisable to drink approximately 1,5 times the weight of the lost liquids, that is 1 liter and ½ every kg of lost weight. Athletes need to intake this amount on a number of occasions until they are completely rehydrated. A rapid replacement of liquids after a physical training restores euhydration, improves recovery, reduces the symptoms of ipohydration and decreases the post-training strain (*Maughan, R. J., Leiper Jb et al., 1995; Maughan, R. J., Leiper Jb et al., 1996*).

It is therefore essential to intake up to 150% of the fluid deficit needed to effectively replace the liquid losses after the physical exercise in a short recovery period (less than 4 hours) (*Institute Of Medicine,2005*). This extra intake is mandatory to compensate the post-training diuresis caused by the fluid load and to restore normal vasopressin hormone levels in the blood. The exact quantity of fluid needed to restore euhydration also depends on the composition of food and on ingestion time after the training, as water and elecrolytes contained in meals contribute to the substitution of fluids and can improve fluid retention (*Leatherwood, W.E.; Dragoo, J.L et al., 2013*). Sports drinks can be more effective than water in speeding up this phase, especially when liquid losses are very high or when athletes must play two rounds in the same day (match play). Intaking water only might lead to a decrease of blood osmolarity (dilution of sodium), reducing the sensation of thirst and increasing diuresis. This might cause a break in the rehydration process before it is complete. Do not forget that skimmed milk is an excellent option for post-competition rehydration, as it improves fluid retention after the physical exercise.

Depending on recovery time, the consumption of meals or snacks with a sufficient amount of water resets euhydration, provided that food contains enough sodium to substitute the perspiration (*Institute Of Medicine,2005)*. In case of relevant dehydration with relatively short recovery time, we can consider more aggressive rehydration programs (*Leatherwood, W.E.; Dragoo, J.L et al., 2013)*. The failure to replace sodium losses inhibits the euhydration and stimulates an excessive production of urine. The consumption of sodium during the recovery time helps retain liquids and stimulates thirst.

7

Nutritional aspects linked to sleep and travel

Professional golfers must travel long distances to take part in the Tour, so they need to be able to manage their nutrition even during these long journeys. It is usually possible to find basic food in most countries, and this allows them not to divert from their standard diet, as unknown local food might be difficult to digest or even hazardous. It is known that travelling many time zones can lead to a deterioration of athletic performances and to an extended recovery time between competitions. Various aspects linked to travelling can influence the athletic performace, but it is difficult to determine to what extent each one plays a role in a sub-optimal performance. We should therefore consider air travelling another stressor, together with competition schedules and training (*Steenland, K.; Deddens, J.A, 1997*), especially when competitions take place within 72 hours of break (*Reilly, T, 2009*). One of the most important consequences is the so-called "travel fatigue".

Travel fatigue is a feeling of disorientation, dizziness, gastrointestinal disorders, impatience, lack of energy and a general discomfort, and it happens after time zone travelling (*Manfredini, R.; Manfredini, F, et al., 1998*). Its extent depends on many circumstances, such as frequency, duration and conditions of the travel.

Specific causes of travel fatigue include jet lag, circadian rhythms interruption, altitude, diet changes, sleep deprivation. There is a damaging effect on athletic performances linked to travelling, caused especially by jet lag, circadian rhythms interruption and the consequent sleep alteration (*Manfredini, R.; Manfredini, F, et al., 1998*). As a matter of fact, circadian rhythm plays a crucial role in sports performances (*Reilly, T.; Waterhouse, J, 2009; Reilly, T.; Waterhouse, J, et al., 2005; Youngstedt, S.D., O'connor, P.J et al., 1999*).

When an athlete's circadian rhythm is syncronized with his environment, the athlete can achieve excellent results (*Youngstedt, S.D., O'connor, P.J et al., 1999*). An plane trip might cause an athlete's circadian rhythm not to be syncronized with the environment anymore (jet lag). As a consequence, the number of time zones plays a fundamental role on the travel fatigue (*Youngstedt, S.D.; O'connor, P.J. et al., 1999; Reilly T., 2009; Loat CE, Rhodes EC, 1989*).

Moreover, it seems that travelling towards East is worse, as far as performances are concerned. This happens because the biological clock is naturally longer than the light-dark cycle of 24 hours, lasting in fact 25-26 hours (*Loat CE, Rhodes EC, 1989*). It is therefore easier for the body to adapt to changes which extend the day instead of shortening it (*Reilly T, Waterhouse J., 2009*).

An alteration of the circadian rhythm, which contributes to the jet lag sensation, affects both the gastrointestinal function and the sleeping pattern (*Reilly T, Waterhouse J., 2009*). The circadian break can cause a delay in the absorption of food in the gastrointestinal tract (*Sanders SW, Moore JG, 1992*). Activity and nutrition schedules change according to the different places, making it hard to adapt to new meals and new activity rhythms. Travelling athletes may also have difficulties find palatable food, which is generally included in their diet. A good meal timing is therefore more important than its energetic income, and small meals before and during the flight are better tolerated than generous ones (*Sanders SW, Moore JG, 1992*). Some foods are particularly important for the resyncronization of the circadian clock. A meal rich in carbs and low in proteins, for instance, can help in absorbing the tryptophan and its convertion in serotonin, inducing drowsiness and sleep. On the other hand, a meal rich in proteins and low in carbs could help the absorption and the conversion of tyrosine in adrenaline, increasing the level of excitement (*Cirelli C, Tononi G, 2008*).

The effect of the changes in the circadian rhythm on sleep is likewise important. Sleep has many physiological and cognitive functions, which are particularly important for top golf players, as well as for other athletes, who can experience a poor quality and/or quantity of sleep (*Cirelli C, Tononi G, 2008*). Sleep deprivation can significantly impact athletic performances, and this is particularly true when it comes to an extended submaximal physical activity such as golf. A chronic and partial deprivation of sleep can also alter the metabolism of carbs, appetite, food intake and protein synthesis.

These elements can ultimately have a negative influence on the nutritional, methabolic and endocrine conditions of the golf player and can potentially reduce athletic performances. The research identified various neurotransmitters associated with the sleep-wake cycle (*Sanders SW, Moore JG. et al, 1992*). All nutritional actions, which can act on these neurotransmitters in the brain, can influence sleep. Carbs, tryptophan, valerian, melatonin, and others, have been studied as potential inducers of sleep, and they represent nutritional aids to be taken into account (*Sanders SW, Moore JG., 1992 et al., 1992*). Post training recovery is vital for athletes, especially for golfers, but if the balance between training stress and physical recovery is insufficient, following performances might be conditioned. An inadequate recovery can reduce the supplies of the autonomic nervous system, jeopardizing the heart rate variability (HRV) and an increase of the resting heart rate (Hynynen, E.S.A.; Uusitalo, A.; *et al, 2006*) (Fig.15)

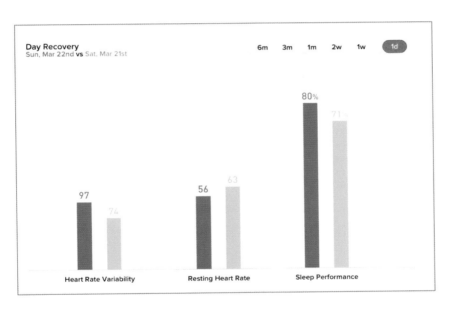

Fig. 15: Heart Rate Variability and Resting Heart Rate related to a deterioration of sleep after an intercontinental flight (Whoop,....)

« *Chrononutrition* » is used to describe the link between food and circadian system (*Tahara, Y.; Shibata, S. et al, 2005*). Our internal clock can be modified changing both the time and nature of food intake (*Tahara, Y.; Shibata, S. et al, 2005*). Sleep can be boosted by inhibiting the mechanisms of wake-promoting effects or increasing sleep-promoting factors through nutritional actions. Nutrients such as antioxidants, tryptophan-rich proteins, carbs, melatonin, micronutrients and fruit can influence sleep (*Shona L. Halson T., 2014*).

Schedules, quantities per meal (large portions and/or late meals in the evening) can negatively influence sleep and therefore circadian rhythms (*Shona L. Halson T., 2014*). Nutrients such as carbs (evening meal with a high glycemic index and reduced latency of sleep-onset), proteins (dairy products can increase the duration of sleep), ethanol (decrease of REM sleep) and caffeine (increase of the latency of sleep-onset, decrease of the total lenght of sleep and decrease of its quality) (*Shona L. Halson T, 2014*). In the same way as diet, also sleeping disorders (problems to start or go on sleeping) and the deprivation of sleep (not sleeping enough time) can be managed to stimulate the recovery and/or the athletic performances (*Venter R.E, 2012*).

To conclude, golf players should definitely focus on a good sleep hygiene to maximise its quality and quantity, but they can also follow other practical recommendations, nutrition included. High glycemic index food, such as white rice, pasta, bread and potatoes can facilitate sleep if they are consumed more than 1 hour before going to sleep. Diets rich in carbs can reduce the latency of sleep, but we should not forget that a decreased total caloric intake can interfere with the quality of sleep. Also diets rich in proteins can improve the quality of sleep, while those rich in fats can negatively influece the rest cycle time (*Peukhuri, K.; Sihvola, N et al., 2012*).

8

Vegetarian Diet

There are many different vegetarian diets, each having a different nutritional values and therefore we need to make a distinction: a vegetarian diet doesn't usually include meat and fish, but eggs, milk, cheese and honey are allowed. Lacto-vegetarian diets leave out eggs. The vegan diet leaves out all foods linked to animals, dairy products included (*Barr SI, Rideout CA, 2004*). As far as sport is concerned, there is no evidence of either good or unhealthy effects, especially if the carbs intake is adequate. Carefully planned vegetarian diets can supply the right energy, thanks to a variety of carbs, fats and proteins, supporting all sports performances. Vegetarian athletes can, in fact, satisfy their need for proteins coming from vegetable sources, if a variety of these foods is consumed daily and the food energy intake is correct (*Barr SI, Rideout CA, 2004; Venderley AM, Campbell WW , 2006; Nieman DC , 1999*).

Even if a vegetarian diet is not linked to harmful effects on athletes, vegetarians need to reach an ideal nutritional intake thanks to a careful planning *(Nieman DC , 1999; Lynch H ,Johnston C, et al., 2018; Phillips SM, Van Loon LJ et al, 2011*). The quality of this intake can be determined in different ways: one of the easiest ones is to measure the ratio of specific nutrients given by the diet itself. Pros and coaches should try to understand the reasons for an athlete's vegetarian choice and correctly train these athletes on how macro- and micronutrients sources can better suit their needs. Coaches should make sure that the player is not disguising an eating disorder with vegetarianism, as it is a psychological problem which can compromise both the athlete's health and athletic performances. Lastly, athletes should never be told that they need to eat animal products to have an adequate nutrition.

Carbs intake is not usually a problem for vegetarian golf players as they mostly have a vegetal origin. Fruit and milk are rich in simple carbs. Refined sugars, such as white sugar, sweets and syrups, are not usually considered a good source of carbs for vegetarians, as they don't provide enough fibers, vitamins or minerals. Complex carbs can easily come from cereals and vegetables. Less refined foods, such as brown rice, whole wheat pasta and bread, are their favourite carbs sources, as they contain more essencial dietary fibres and B-group vitamins. Even though a typical vegetarian diet is rich in carbs, it is important to take enough quantity, especially if we think about how popular low carbs diets have become, and how attractive they can be for some vegetarian golfers. These can easily satisfy their energy needs with foods rich in fats, such as nuts and seeds, olives, olive oil, sesame oil and avocado. On the other hand it is common to find vegetarian athletes on diets, which are too rich in saturated fats mainly coming from low-fats dairy products. Health benefits can come from a strict vegetarian diet, with a fat intake lower than 10%, while a serious limitation in fats can harm ideal athletic performances, particularly for athletes engaged in prolongued training or in subsequent competitions with no rest. Vegetarian golfers can have the right fats intake thanks to a careful selection of plant-based sources and of low-fat dairy products. Generally speaking, the vegetarian diet is rich in omega-6 polyunsaturated fatty acids, but it also poor in omega-3 fatty acids (*Phillips SM, Van Loon LJ et al, 2011).*

Vegetarian athletes can easily get not only the right intake of proteins with plant protein foods, such as legumes, cereals, nuts and seeds, but also all the essential and non essential amino acids, if their diet is varied. A well-planned vegetarian diet should include, on average, 12.5% of energy coming from proteins. (*Lynch H ,Johnston C, et al., 2018).* We don't have enough evidence that protein requirements are different, if athletes are on a vegetarian diet. Vegetarian athletes should be encouraged to eat a range of foods rich in plant-based proteins, if they want to be sure about an ideal proteins intake. It is important to remember that all cereals and starchy vegetables contain a small amount of proteins. Vegetarians should therefore eat a variety of protein sources throughout the day, rather than eating particular mixes of plant-based proteins every meal. This is always true, except for post-training periods, to optimize muscle protein synthesis (*Lynch H ,Johnston C, et al., 2018*). Protein food combinations, such as rice and beans, beans and nuts or a peanut butter sandwich, can be, for instance, complementary.

8. 1 Supplements in the vegetarian diet

8.1.1 Creatine

When considering athletic performances, you need to remember that creatine concentrations are lower in vegetarian athletes compared to non vegetarian ones (*Lukaszuk JM, Robertson RJ, et al., 2005*). The estimated daily need is 2 grams. Non vegetarians usually get 1 gram of creatine per day from meat, being the rest synthesised, mainly in the liver. We have evidence that an inadequate intake of creatine coming from meat is not compensated by an increase in the endogenous production of it (*Williams MH, Branch JD, 1998; Bemben MG, Lamont HS., 2005*). Vegetarian athletes should be conscious of what it means to have a lower pool of creatine in their body, compared to non vegetarian counterparts. It is therefore reasonable to suggest them creatine supplementation.

8.1.2 Iron

In a vegetarian diet iron is absorbed in the form of non heme-iron, which has a relatively low absorption rate (2-20%) compared to heme-iron (15-35%) eaten with meat (*Chiplonkar SA, Agte VV, 2006*). In addition to that, some substances of vegetable origins, such as bran, polyphenols, egg yolk, soy beans products and phytic acid can interfere with the absorption of iron (*Hunt JR, 2003*). A low iron intake and a reduced absorption can therefore reduce iron stored in vegetarian golfers. In most cases they can meet the appropriate iron quantity with no iron supplements, if they avoid foods which interfere with the absorption, and they increase the intake of substances, known to increase non heme-iron absorption, such as vitamin C, citric acid, malic acid, tartaric acid, fructose and sorbitol. High dose iron supplements should not be taken, unless blood test show an iron deficiency.

It is important to underline that zinc and iron supplements should not include more than 100% of the recommended dietary allowance, to avoid negative interactions with the absorption of other nutrients (*Hunt JR, 2003*). Like iron, a sub-optimal level of zinc can be somehow dominant in some athletes, including female athletes on vegan and vegetarian diets. A low level of zinc in vegetarians can be linked to a selection of food low in zinc or to its reduced bioavailability in plants compared to foods of animal origin. Vegetarians, whose diet is varied and balanced, with many foods rich in zinc, including legumes and whole-grain cereals, will probably reach a good level of zinc with no dietary supplements.

8.1.3 Vitamins

Vegetarian diets can satisfy most of vitaminic needs, except for vitamin B12, vitamin D and vitamin B2. B2 is necessary for many cellular processes and, as the other B group vitamins, plays a key role in the energy metabolism. The dietary intake of B2 can be limited in vegetarian diets, especially if you abstain from soy milk and soy milk based products. Vegetarian athletes, especially if they avoid dairy products, sould be taught how to increase their intake of plant sources of B2, such as cereals, soy seeds, soy milk, almonds, asparagus, bananas, sweet potatoes and wheat germ.

No plant food has vitamin D, and you can find it in very few foods, all of animal origin, such as fish, liver, eggs and dairy food. Vitamin D is synthesised in the skin by exposure to sunlight and this synthesis is usually good in golf players, who reach overall conditions during summer months in temperate areas and all year round in equatiorial regions. Vegetarian athletes with insufficient sunlight exposure, including those who cover their skin for religious or cultural reasons, or whose skin is dark, are at risk of vitamin D deficiency. In such cases, you should take fortified foods or supplements to ensure adequate levels of it.

Vitamin B12 plays a key role in maintaining the normal function of the nervous system and of blood *(Ryan-Harshman M, Aldoori W, 2008)*, in processing fat acids and in the production of energy *(Woolf K, Manore MM, 2006)*. Vegetarian golfers who eat eggs, cheese, milk and yoghurt get an adequate amount of it. On the other hand, those who are on stricter diets need to eat vitamin B12 fortified foods or supplements on a regular basis. A well-balanced vegetarian diet usually provides an abundance of other nutrients, such as potassium, magnesium, folic acids, vitamins A, C, E, and K *(Woolf K, Manore MM, 2006)*.

9

Vegan Diet

Over the past few years, professional athletes, including golf players, have been experiencing vegan diet. This is a sort of vegetarianism, which bans animal products, and, as is known, has proven to have many health benefits. An increase in fruit, vegetables and whole-grain cereals can help the weight management, thanks to a better digestion, restful sleep and can reduce the risk of heart diseases, type II diabetes, hypertension and some cancers (*Melina, V., Craig W, et al., 1980; Fuhrman J, Ferreri DM, 2010*). Vegan diet can bring potential benefits to sports performances, thanks to the consumption of foods rich in carbs, typical of plant-based diets, antioxidants (polyphenols) and micronutrients (vitamins C, E), which help the training performance and enhance recovery (*Craddock, J.C., Y.C. Probst et al., 2016; Nieman, D.C, 1988*). Completetly abolishing foods of animal origin in a golfer's diet is not always the healthier choice, if it is not correctly performed. Even though many vegan restaurants are now open, there are many places, including restaurants in golf clubs, that have not kept up with the times. This means that it is difficult, also from a practical point of view, to stick to a vegan diet.

Data suggest that vegans usually use less energy than omnivores, and that vegan diets are low in proteins, fats, vitamin B12, riboflavin, vitamin D, calcium, iron and zinc compared to an omnivorous diet (*Clarys P, Deliens T, et al, 2018*). An insufficient calories intake can forfeit the benefits of the training, compromise performances and can lead to health complications (loss of muscle mass and / or of bone density), with an increased risk of fatigue, injuries and illnesses, particularly for a golf player. Managing the energy balance is therefore fundamental, even if it can be even worse when the diet gives early satiety and reduced appetite, as it happens with the vegan diet (Craddock, J.C., Y.C. Probst et al., 2016; Clarys P, Deliens T, et al, 2018). If you need a rich in calories diet, you should, for example, increase the frequency both of meals and foods rich in energy, such as nuts, seeds and oils, thus being able to reach calorie goals. Diet monitoring and adjusting according to fluctuations in body weight could also help adapt the diet to the player's energy and nutritional needs (Rogerson D, 2017). Apparently vegan athletes eat less proteins than their omnivore and vegetarian counterparts. The non-optimization of the intake of proteins for these athletes calls for attention as far as quantity and quality of proteins eaten. Plant-sources proteins are often incomplete, they lack important essential amino acids, and they usually contain less branched-chain amino acids compared to their animal-based counterparts (*Clarys P, Deliens T, et al, 2018*). Foods such as cereals, legumes, nuts and seeds should be included in the vegan diet, to guarantee the intake of all essential amino acids and an adequate amount of branched-chain ones to help the recovery and the adaptation to the training session. Additional proteins could be of interest to vegan golfers, particularly if achieving adequate amounts of proteins with whole-grain foods is difficult or less viable.

Vegan diets tend to be richer in carbs, fibers, fruit, vegetables, antioxidants and phytochemicals compared to omnivore diets, and the intake of micronutrients and foods rich in phytochemicals is a significant aspect for any plant-based diet (Clarys P, Deliens T, et al, 2018). It is relatively easy to reach the right intake of carbs with a vegan diet. Cereals, legumes, beans, tubers, root vegetables and fruit can all be eaten to adequately meet needs of carbs. We recommend vegans to eat beans, legumes, lentils and cereals, foods that are all rich in carbs, on a daily basis, to be able to reach sufficient protein amounts with whole-grain foods.

Vegan diets are usually low in total fat and in saturated fat and richer in Omega-6 fats, compared to omnivore and vegetarian diets (*Clarys P, Deliens T, et al, 2018*). Reaching the recommended level (20% of the daily calory intake) is possible for vegan athletes with the right consumption of oils, avocado, nuts and seeds.

A vegan diet can fulfill the needs of most golfers, if there is a strategic selection and a management of food choices, a particular focus on reaching energy recommendations of macro and micro nutrients, together with the right supplements *(Woo KS, Kwok CYT et al., 2014)*. A pre-round meal, which, as you know, should end about 3 hours in advance, to give our body the time to digest food, should include carbs rich in low glycemic index fibers, such as oat, to ensure a gradual release of energy in the upcoming hours. This baseline needs to be completed with other dietary high-quality fat sources, to provide low intensity fuel. Examples are nuts, seeds, avocado, etc. and some fruit and/or vegetables to increase the content of micronutrients in the meal.

The aim of the vegan diet in a competition is the same of the omnivore diet: keep settled energy levels and keep hydrated to maximise mental focus. As a results, snacks have a similar trend, aiming to supply with low glycemic index carbs, a small quantity of proteins and some high quality fats. To secure a constant supply of energy and reduce the symptoms of hunger, it is better to evenly distribute 3-4 snacks during the round.

10

Supplements

An ergogenic support is any ingredient or nutrition practice that can improve the performance of the exercise or the training adaptations. Nutritional aids can help a person prepare for physical exercise, improve exercise effectiveness and recovery or help prevent injuries during an intensive training (*Kreider RB, Wilborn CD et al., 2010*). This might seem easy, but there is a significate debate on the ergogenic value of many supplements. You can call food supplement ergogenic, if peer-review studies show that it considerably improves performances after weeks or months of ingestion (for example, it increases maximum strength, running speed and or speed of work during a particular exercise). On the other hand, a supplement can have an ergogenic value, if it sharply improves the athlete's ability to perform a physical activity or his recovery after a single training session.

A proper nutritional plan, inspired by the above-mentioned simple principles, is usually enough to totally cover nutritional needs of almost all sportspeople. The need for supplements is often unnecessary and not completely risk-free for the health, even if only potential, as some of these products may include toxic substances and/or are included in the list of doping substances.

Sports supplements include a wide and varied range of products (minerals, vitamins, energetic nutrients, plant extracts, amino acids, etc.) and they are usually on the market to compensate for deficiencies in one or more nutrients, caused by inadequate intake with the normal diet. Most supplements used in sport are usually contained in food (amino acids, creatine, L-Carnitine, caffeine, etc.) and marketed as « extracts » or industrially synthesised. Many of the advertised effects are just alleged, and this is shown by a few studies, well checked and correctly carried out, on many of these alleged nutritional ergogenic substances. You need to carefully evaluate the use of ergogenic products, not forgetting that a contamination with banned substances not listed on the label, such as steroids or other banned stimulants, is always possible.

The peculiarity of golf activity leads us to focus on three substances, which we can successfully use : caffeine, antioxidants and probiotics.

10.1 Caffeine

Caffeine has both physiological and psychological effects and it has become one of the most common ergogenic aids in professional golf.

Benefits of caffeine are not limited exclusively to a physical performance improvement, as various studies show its effectiveness in improving cognitive performances (*Kennedy DO, Scholey AB, 2004*) as well as the physically demanding ones (*Smit H, Rogers P, 2000*). As professional golf requires high cognitive and motor performances, fatigue can negatively impact on results through both central and peripheral mechanisms.

The fatigue retardant effect of caffeine is well known, as it acts stimulating the central nervous system mainly thanks to its interactions with adenosine receptors, increasing the exitability of the neuronal tissue. It has been proven that consuming moderate quantities of caffeine (100-300 mg) has a positive effect on cognitive and motor performances during sports activities (*Hogervorst E, Bandelow S et al., 2008*). A moderate quantity reduces the golfer's specific fatigue, and it seems to lead to greater precision and overall better performances (*Mumford PW1, Tribby AC et al., 2016*).

The ideal quantity should be the smallest possible (1-3 mg/kg), to avoid side effects. We should not forget that the average caffeine content per espresso is 50-100 mg, per tea cup is 40 mg and per cola drink is 40 mg. Threshold plasma concentrations needed to have an ergogenic answer can vary, if the intake of caffeine happens before the exercise (higher) or during the exercise (lower). These threshold concentrations happen to be lower for non-regular caffeine users compared to regular consumers and the ergogenic response is present for some hours after the intake. When scheduling the intake, we need to remember that the plasma peak comes about 60-90 minutes after the consumption, and that its plasma concentration is halved after about 2-3 hours (Fig.16).

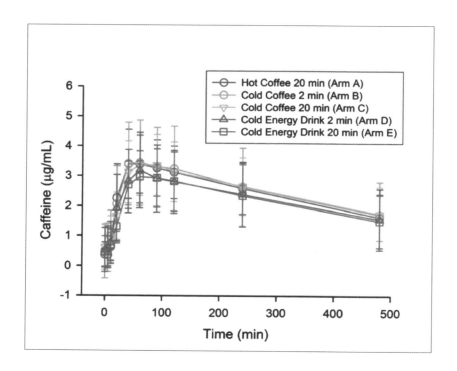

Fig. 16: Pharmakokinetics of caffeine after an oral administration of different formulations (from: White JR, Padowski JM, Zhong Y, Chen G, Luo S, Lazarus P, Layton ME, McPherson S. Pharmacokinetic analysis and comparison of caffeine administered rapidly or slowly in coffee chilled or hot versus chilled energy drink in healthy young adults. Clin Toxicol, 2016; 54, (4): 308–312).

There are substantial differences in individual responses to caffeine. In addition to that, very high quantities (6 or more mg per kg) can degrade both physical and cognitive performances, as they can lead to anxiety and severe gastrointestinal disorders. These individual responses show that players should always test the effects of caffeine on themselves before a competition, to be able to optimise the dose, ingestion time, and the period of abstinence before the competition. They should also check on an increased resting heart rate, tremors, over-exitation, fine motor skills disorders (Fig. 17). Some people are more susceptible than others, which means that, in case of these side effects, it is better to avoid its use (*Smit H, Rogers P, 2000*).

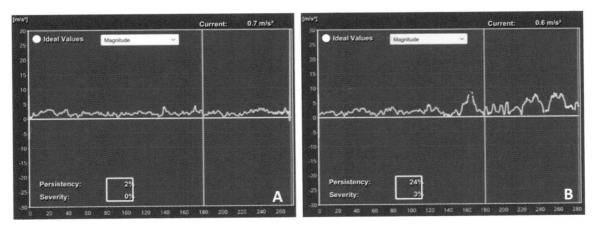

Fig.17: evaluation of tremor during the putting after an intake of 500 mg of caffeine (B) and in normal conditions (A) (Sistema CAPTO, Arezzo, Italy)

10.2 Antioxidants

It is known that sports workout can increase free radicals in oxygen. Once they overcome the antioxidant capacity of the body, they can cause inflammation, muscle weakness and fatigue. Golf practice involves an alternation of multiple muscle contractions (walking) and explosive movements (swing). These can cause a muscle overload at different levels, according not only to the intensity and the duration of the activity, but also to the player's training status. Antioxidants can reduce the combined effects of training sessions and competitions on the physiological and physical function. A key category for antioxidants are polyphenols, a wide range of natural, plant-derived compounds (*Duthie GG, Gardner PT, et al., 2003*), which are usually included in the list of supplements intended for sports use.

The results of several studies show that the use of polyphenols, both close to a competition (acute) and in the weeks leading up to it (chronic), is linked to an improvement of performances without any negative side effects, and that it plays a role in the recovery of muscle function after the training (*Bowtell J, Kelly G, 2019*).

Fruit, vegetables and fruit-derived polyphenols supplements contain a variable mixture of polyphenols. Intersubject bioavailability will therefore be different in each case, due to the differences in the intestinal microbiome, which plays a role in activating them (*Kay CD, Pereira-Caro G et al., 2017; Crozier A, Del Rio D et al., 2010*). Many natural polyphenols are in fact characterized by a low intestinal absorption in the human being, and this reduced bioavailabilty itself is a serious limitation to the potential beneficial effects of these compounds (*Crozier A, Del Rio D et al., 2010*).

Polyphenols are biotransformed into active compounds by the intestinal microbiota itself, thus acquiring a bigger intestinal absorption and a better bioavailabilty. Thanks to the biotransformation run by the microbiome, they can reach the bloodstream more easily and exercise their biologically relevant effects systemically (*Seeram NP, Zhang Y et al., 2008*). The increase of the blood concentration of polyphenols is evident within 30 minutes from ingestion, with concentrations of metabolites peaks within 1-2 hours (*Crum EM, Muhamed AMC et al., 2017*).

The time of intake is consequently a key point. All the studies, where the intake of supplements took place within 1 hour from the training, showed clear ergogenic effects ; on the other hand, when the intake took place more that 2 hour before, the performances did not improve (*Crum EM, Muhamed AMC et al., 2017*).

In conclusion, present evicende tell us that acute integration with about 300 mg of polyphenols 1 hour before the exercise can be ergogenic, while the integration with more than 1000 mg of polyphenols per day for 3 days or more before and after the exercise will improve the recovery after sports events which can lead to tissue damage. This happens with sports such as golf, where you have many rounds in a row and short recovery times. The intake of 450g of blueberries, 120g of blackcurrants or 300g of cherries could approximately result in this amount.

10.3 Probiotics

Human gut contains a rich and diversified microbial ecosystem, whose activities can affect our health. To be more precise, our intestine hosts trillions of microbial species (*Janssens,*

Y.; Nielandt, J et al., 2018), which coexist with human cells.

This collection of microbes is called microbiota. Despite the fact that microbiota is stable in adults, several factors, such as age, genetics, drugs, stress, smoke and diet, can influence it, modifying a complex, highly dynamic and individual ecosystem (*Gill, S.R.; Pop, M et al 2006*). Athletes in general, including golf players, have different compositions of intestinal microbiota, which seem to reflect the level of physical exercise compared to sedentary people. These differences are mainly linked to the amount of training and to the quantity of proteins in the diet (*Barton, W.; Penney, N.C et al., 2017*).

A prolongued and intense physical exercise, such as a training session or a competition, generate a state of stress on the gastrointestinal tract, increasing the probability of multiple symptoms associated with an alterated intestinal microbiota. This includes abdominal cramps, acid reflux (heartburn), nausea, vomit, diarrhea, all linked to reduced performances (*Clarke, S.F.; Murphy, E.F et al., 2014*).

There is also another link, typical of golf, between physical and emotional stress during physical exercise and changes in the composition of intestinal microbiota. An alterated microbioma can influence the energy metabolism, the immune function, and the oxidative stress. These are all vital elements for the athlete's performance and for health in general (*Mach, N.; Fuster-Botella, D. et al., 2017*). Diet is a consolidated modulator in the composition of intestinal microbiota, with a significant change recorded within 24 hours from a diet change (*Karl, J.P.; Margolis, L.M et al., 2017*). Many food components, diet schemes and nutrients can dramatically alter the growth of different microbial populations. Protein intake seems to be a strong modular of macrobiota variety, and whey proteins show some potential benefits (*Clarke, S.F.; Murphy, E.F et al., 2014*). Also higher intakes of carbs and dietary fibres in athletes seems to be associated with an increase and a diversification of useful intestinal microbial populations. Specific effects of fat on the intestinal microbiota are, on the other hand, difficult to evaluate, but it seems that all fats are important.

Due to the high complexity of élite golfers' responses to stress, it is difficult to define standard diets. What concerns us, is that dietary recommendations for them are largely based on a low intake of plan polysaccharides, which reflects on a reduced diversity and functionality of the microbiota. They are usually recommended appropriate nutritional choices (that is, avoiding fats and fibers) to reduce the risk of gastrointestinal discomfort, ensuring a rapid gastric emptying, water and nutrients absorption and an adequate perfusion of the splanchnic vascular system before the competitions. A lack of complex carbs in élite athletes' diets can nonetheless negatively influence the composition and the functioning of the intestinal microbiota in the long run. The intake of complex plant polysaccharides should therefore be encouraged, to be able to keep the diversity and the function of the intestinal microbiota. It is also to be noticed that a high intake of animal proteins during their days of rest and training should be reduced, as they could negatively influence the intestinal microbiota (*Jäger et al., 2019*).

In addition to the above mentioned dietary advice, another way to keep the microbiota healthy is probiotics. Probiotics are living bacteria, which confer a benefit to the hosting body, when they are orally consumed in an adequante quantity for some weeks (*Jäger et al., 2019*). Supplementing your diet with probiotics, which stimulate the expansion of specific microorganisms to improve the metabolic, immune and barrier functions, can be a real therapy for golf players. In this sense, the modulation of microbiota and its fermentation ability can give scientific basis to plan diets, which are focused on boosting performances, improving the metabolites of the healthy microbiota during the exercise while limiting those who produce toxic metabolites, as the latter might deteriorate stress cosequences. Probiotic supplementation varies according to the strain and to the composition of the microbiota. This means that there are no specific dietary recommendations, as far as doses or strains for golfers are concerned (*Wosinska L, Cotter PD et al., 2019*).

An analysis of the intestinal microbiota would help to get a useful picture to plan our dietary or supplementation choices (Fig.18)

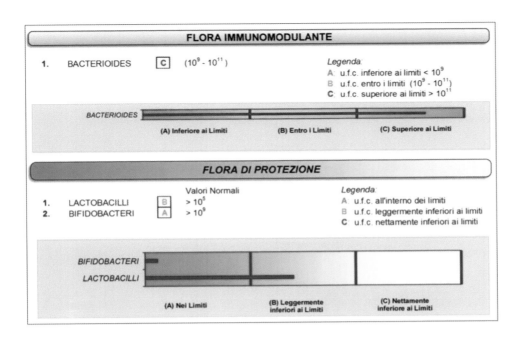

Fig. 18: Analysis of the intestinal microbiota.

Like other dietary supplements, we should consider probiotics as part of a balanced diet. Nutritional needs should always be fulfilled by a « food first » approach, that is eating whole foods rather than supplements (*Jäger R, Mohr AE, et al., 2019*). It's also important to remember that some probiotic foods, such as yoghurt, include energy, carbs, proteins and other nutrients that can be part of a golfer's nutritional plan. There are different formulations on the market to meet individual tastes. Some are tablets or capsule in powder form, to be added to drinks, others are chewable tablets rich in probiotics.

More and more supplements with probiotics are on the market around the world. The strains of probiotics show specific differences when focusing on their capacity to colonise the gastrointestinal tract, their clinical efficacy, the type and entity of health benefits in a range of different cohorts of the population. The majority of probiotics strains is traditionally represented by the group of lactic acid bacteria, that is Bifidobacterium, Lactobacillus. However, other bacterial and yeast strains, such as Escherichia coli e Saccharomyces, are commonly used (*Santosa, S.; Farnworth, E, 2006; Ramos, C.L.; Thorsen, L.;et al., 2013*). One of the main concerns about this market is that some strains have shown no substantial evidence. Players should also be aware that the benefits of one probiotic strain cannot be obtained from another one. Technology led to probiotic supplements which do not need refrigeration, and these can be suitable for golf players, when travelling.

On a practical level, a golfer should start consuming probiotic supplements at least 14 days before an intensive training session or an important competition, to give them the right time for the transient colonization or for the bacterial species to adapt. Another important issue is the increasing risk of gastrointestinal problems during their trips (*Jeukendrup AE, Vet-Joop K et al 2000*). Probiotics supplementation for travelling individuals and athletes could be part of a comprehensive plan of disease prevention.

The players' tolerance and side effects should always be monitored, because they can experience an increase in the intestinal transition activities during the colonization period. These include rumbling gut, flatulence increase, etc. Athletes should be informed that mild side effects may occur for some days (*Santosa, S.; Farnworth, E, 2006).*

It is advisable to test probiotics supplementation during both offseason and preseason periods, so that the golf player can become familiar with the assumption before either the trip or the competition and can check his responses. This is also useful when evaluating individual tolerance and potential side effects.

11

Nutrition Plans

GOLF ROUND NUTRITION PLAN – 1

GRAMS

KCAL

	Night before	> 3 hours pre	> 1 hour pre	During (every 15 min)	Post (within 1 hour)
Carbs	44,8	118	39,5	4,6	101
Proteins	30,7	48	11	0,3	46,6
Fats	38,3	9,3	6	0,09	29
kcal	773	719	100	20	825

- Night before: Homemade beef burger on a whole wheat bun with lettuce, tomato and sauce
- > 3 hours pre: Wholewheat spaghetti with turkey meatballs in a tomato sauce with broccoli
- > 1 hour pre: Chopped banana on a crumpet
- During (every 15 min): Handfull of dried bananas
- Post (within 1 hour): Egg noodles with salmon, broccoli and cheese sauce

GOLF ROUND NUTRITION PLAN– 2

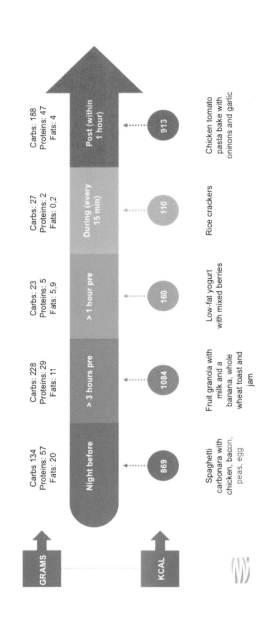

	Night before	> 3 hours pre	> 1 hour pre	During (every 15 min)	Post (within 1 hour)
GRAMS	Carbs 134 Proteins: 57 Fats: 20	Carbs: 228 Proteins: 29 Fats: 11	Carbs: 23 Proteins: 5 Fats: 5,9	Carbs: 27 Proteins: 2 Fats: 0,2	Carbs: 188 Proteins: 47 Fats: 4
KCAL	869	1084	160	110	913
	Spaghetti carbonara with chicken, bacon, peas, egg	Fruit granola with milk and a banana, whole wheat toast and jam	Low-fat yogurt with mixed berries	Rice crackers	Chicken tomato pasta bake with oninons and garlic

GOLF ROUND NUTRITION PLAN– 3

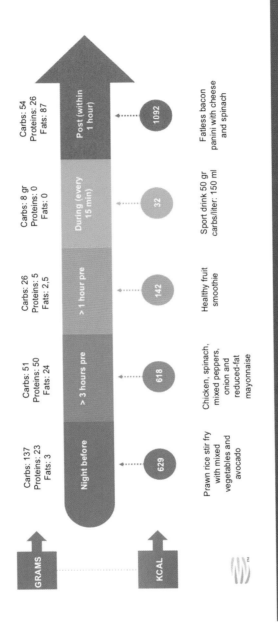

GRAMS

KCAL

	Night before	> 3 hours pre	> 1 hour pre	During (every 15 min)	Post (within 1 hour)
Macros	Carbs: 137 Proteins: 23 Fats: 3	Carbs: 51 Proteins: 50 Fats: 24	Carbs: 26 Proteins: 5 Fats: 2.5	Carbs: 8 gr Proteins: 0 Fats: 0	Carbs: 54 Proteins: 26 Fats: 87
Kcal	629	618	142	32	1092
Food	Prawn rice stir fry with mixed vegetables and avocado	Chicken, spinach, mixed peppers, onion and reduced-fat mayonnaise	Healthy fruit smoothie	Sport drink 50 gr carbs/liter: 150 ml	Fatless bacon panini with cheese and spinach

12

QUESTIONAIRE ON EATING HABITS

Surname:
Name:
Age:

Weight:
Height:

Training

	< 1 /week	Up to 3/week	> 3/week	Every day
Gym	☐	☐	☐	☐
Driving range	☐	☐	☐	☐
18 holes	☐	☐	☐	☐

Where do you usually eat your meals?

	HOME	CANTEEN	FAST-FOOD	RESTAURANT	OTHER
Breakfast	☐	☐	☐	☐	☐
Morning break	☐	☐	☐	☐	☐
Lunch	☐	☐	☐	☐	☐
Break	☐	☐	☐	☐	☐
Dinner	☐	☐	☐	☐	☐

SPECIFIC DIET	YES☐ NO☐	
GLUTEN INTOLERANCE	YES☐ NO☐	
FOOD ALLERGIES OR INTOLERANCES	YES☐ NO☐	

FOOD SUPPLEMENTS	☐ YES
FREQUENCY OF CONSUMPTION	☐ REGULAR
TYPE OF SUPPLEMENT	☐ VITAMINS
	☐ MINERALS
	☐ VITAMINS AND MINERALS
	☐ PROTEINS/AMINO ACIDS
	☐ FIBERS
	☐ ANTIOXIDANTS
	☐ PROBIOTICS

Frequency of consumption	YEAR	DAY	WEEK	MONTH	NEVER
CEREALS AND CEREAL PRODUCTS (pasta,rice, pizza, spelt, barley)	☐	☐	☐	☐	☐
CEREAL-BASED PRODUCTS (cornflakes, biscuits, rusks, saltines)	☐	☐	☐	☐	☐
FRESH MEAT	☐	☐	☐	☐	☐
PROCESSED MEAT (ham, salami, cured meats)	☐	☐	☐	☐	☐
FISH	☐	☐	☐	☐	☐
MILK AND JOGHURT	☐	☐	☐	☐	☐
FRESH AND MATURE CHEESE	☐	☐	☐	☐	☐
FRESH FRUIT	☐	☐	☐	☐	☐
DRIED FRUIT	☐	☐	☐	☐	☐
VEGETABLES	☐	☐	☐	☐	☐
LEGUMES (beans, lentils, peas, chickpeas)	☐	☐	☐	☐	☐
EGGS	☐	☐	☐	☐	☐
SWEETS	☐	☐	☐	☐	☐
SOFT DRINKS	☐	☐	☐	☐	☐
ALCOHOLIC DRINKS	☐	☐	☐	☐	☐

BIBLIOGRAPHY

Ainsworth B., Haskell, W.L., Whitt M.C. et al, (2000). Compendium of physical activities: an update of activity codes and MET intensities. Med Sci Sports Exerc.32:S498–S504

American College of Sports Medicine [ACSM] (2009). ACSM's guidelines for exercise testing and prescription. 8th ed. Williams & Wilkins, New York

American College of Sports Medicine, American Dietetic Association, Dietitians of Canada. Joint Position Statement: nutrition and athletic performance. American College of Sports Medicine, American Dietetic Association, Dietitians of Canada. (2000). Med Sci Sports Exerc 32(12):2130–45.

Atkinson FS, Foster-Powell K, Brand-Miller JC (2008). International tables of glycemic index and glycemic load values: Diabetes Care. 31(12):2281-3.

Barr SI, Rideout CA. Nutritional considerations for vegetarian athletes. (2004). Nutrition 20: 696-703

Barton, W.; Penney, N.C.; Cronin, O.; Garcia-Perez, I.; Molloy, M.G.; Holmes, E.; Shanahan, F.; Cotter, P.D.; O'Sullivan, O. (2017). The microbiome of professional athletes differs from that of more sedentary subjects in composition and particularly at the functional metabolic level. Gut 67, 625–633

Bean A. (2013). The complete guide to sport nutrition. Bloomsbury Publishing, London

Bemben MG, Lamont HS. (2005). Creatine supplementation and exercise performance: recent findings. Sports Med 35:107-125

Bergeron, M.F.; Bahr, R.; Bartsch, P.; Bourdon, L.; Calbet, J.A.L.; Carlsen, K.H.; Castagna, O.; González-Alonso, J.; Lundby, C.; Maughan, R.J.; et al. (2012). International Olympic Committee consensus statement on thermoregulatory and altitude challenges for high-level athletes. Br. J. Sports Med. 46, 770–779.

Bowtell j, Kelly G. (2019). Fruit-Derived Polyphenol Supplementation for Athlete Recovery and Performance . Sports Medicine 49 (Suppl 1):S3–S23

Burke L, Heeley P. Dietary supplements and nutritional ergogenic aids in sport. In: Burke L, Deakin V, editors. Clinical sports nutrition. Sydney, Australia: McGraw-Hill Book Company

Burke L. (2011). Carbohydrates for training and competition J. Sports Sci 29(1): 17-27

Burke L. (2007). Pratical Sports Nutrition, Human Kinetics, Champaign, IL

Burke, L.M., Close, G.L., Lundy, B., Mooses, M., Morton, J.PTenforde, A.S. (2018). Relative energy deficiency in sport in male athletes: A commentary on its presentation among selected groups of male athletes. International Journal of Sport Nutrition and Exercise Metabolism 28(4), 364–374

Burkett LN, von Heijne-Fisher U. Heart rate and calorie expenditure of golfers carrying their clubs and walking flat and hilly golf courses. (1998). International Sports Journal 2:78–85.

Castro-Sepúlveda M, Cerda-Kohler H, Pérez-Luco C, Monsalves M, Cristobal D, HZbinden-FonceaH, Báez-San Martín E, Ramírez-Campillo R. (2015). Hydration status after exercise affect resting metabolic rate and heart rate variability Nutr Hosp. 31(3):1273-1277

Cheuvront SN, Kenefick RW. (2014). Dehydration: physiology, assessment, and performance effects. Compr Physiol. 4(1):257-85

Cheuvront, S.N.; Kenefick, R.W. (2016). Am I Drinking Enough? Yes, No, and Maybe. J. Am. Coll. Nutr. 35, 185–192.

Chiplonkar SA, Agte VV. (2006). Statistical model for predicting non-heme iron bioavailability from vegetarian meals. Int J Food Sci Nutr 57: 434-450.

Cirelli C, Tononi G. (2008). Is sleep essential? PLoS Biol. 6(8): e216.

Clarke, S.F.; Murphy, E.F.; O'Sullivan, O.; Lucey, A.J.; Humphreys, M.; Hogan, A.; Hayes, P.; O'Reilly, M.; Jeffery, I.B.; Wood-Martin, R.; et al. (2014). Exercise and associated dietary extremes impact on gut microbial diversity. Gut 63, 1913–1920.

Clarys P, Deliens T, Huybrechts I, Deriemaeker P, Vanaelst B, De Keyzer W, et al. (2014). Comparison of nutritional quality of the vegan, vegetarian, semi-vegetarian, pesco-vegetarian and omnivorous diet. Nutrients. 6(3):1318–32.

Coggan AR, Coyle EF (2011). Carbohydrate ingestion during prolonged exercise: effect on metabolism and performance, in J. Holloszy Exercise and Sports Science Reviews, vol 19 William and Wilkins pp 1-40.

Coyle E (2004). Fluid and fuel intake during exercise. J Sports Sci 22: 39-55

Coyle EF (1988). Carbohydrates and athletic performance. Sports Sci Exch Sports Nutr Gatorade Sports Science Institute, Vol. 1

Craddock J.C., Y.C. Probst, and G.E. Peoples (2016). Vegetarian and omnivorous nutrition - comparing physical performance. Int. J. Sport Nutr. Exerc. Metab. 26:212-220.

Crozier A, Del Rio D, Clifford MN. (2010). Bioavailability of dietary flavonoids and phenolic compounds. Mol Aspects Med. 31(6):446–67.

Crum EM, Muhamed AMC, Barnes M, Stannard SR. (2017). The effect of acute pomegranate extract supplementation on oxygen uptake in highly-trained cyclists during high-intensity exercise in a high altitude environment. J Int Soc Sports Nutr. 14:14

Dinu M., R. Abbate, G.F. Gensini, A. Casini, and F. Sofi (2017). Vegetarian, vegan diets and multiple health outcomes: a systematic review with meta-analysis of observational studies. Crit. Rev. Food Sci. Nutr. 57:3640-3649.

Duthie GG, Gardner PT, Kyle JAM. Plant polyphenols: are they the new magic bullet? Proc Nutr Soc. 2003;62(3):599–603.

Fuhrman J, Ferreri DM. Fueling the vegetarian (vegan) athlete. Curr Sports ⸤SEP⸥Med Rep. 2010;9(4):233–41

Gammone MA, Riccioni G, Parrinello G, D'Orazio N. Omega-3 Polyunsaturated Fatty Acids: Benefits and Endpoints in Sport. Nutrients. 2018 Dec 27;11(1): E46

Gill, S.R.; Pop, M.; DeBoy, R.T.; Eckburg, P.B.; Turnbaugh, P.J.; Samuel, B.S.; Gordon, J.I.; Relman, D.A.; Fraser-Liggett, C.M.; Nelson, K.E. Metagenomic analysis of the human distal gut microbiome. Science 2006, 312, 1355–1359 ⸤SEP⸥

Hao, L., Chen, Q., Lu, J.; Li, Z.; Guo, C.; Ping Qian, P.; Jianyong Yua, J.; Xing, X. A novel hypotonic sports drink containing a high molecular weight polysaccharide. Food Funct. 2014, 5, 961

Haugen HA, Chan LN, Li F. Indirect Calorimetry: A Practical Guide for Clinicians. Nutr Clin Pract. 2007 Aug;22(4):377-88

Hills PA , Mokhtar N, Byrne NM. Assessment of Physical Activity and Energy Expenditure: An Overview of Objective Measures. Front. Nutr., 2014; 5: 1-6

Hogervorst E, Bandelow S, Schmitt J, et al. Caffeine improves physical and cognitive performance during exhaustive exercise. Med Sci Sports Exerc. 2008;40(10):1841–51.

Howarth KR, Moreau NA, Phillips SM, Gibala MJ. Coingestion Of Protein With Carbohydrate During Recovery From Endurance Exercise Stimulates Skeletal Muscle Protein Synthesis In Humans. J Appl Physiol. 2009;106(4):1394–402.

Hunt JR. . Bioavailability of iron, zinc, and other trace minerals from vegetarian diets. Am J Clin Nutr 2003; 78(3 Suppl): 633S-639S.

Hynynen, E.S.A.; Uusitalo, A.; Konttinen, N.; Rusko, H. Heart rate variability during night sleep and after awakening in overtrained athletes. Med. Sci. Sports Exerc. 2006, 38, 313–317.

Institute Of Medicine. Water. In: Dietary Reference Intakes for Water, Sodium, Cholride, Potassium and Sulfate, Washington, D.C: National Academy Press, pp. 73–185, 2005.

Jäger et al. International Society of Sports Nutrition Position Stand: protein and exercise . Journal of the International Society of Sports Nutrition (2017) 14:20

Jäger et al. International Society of Sports Nutrition Position Stand: Probiotics Journal of the International Society of Sports Nutrition (2019) 16:62-85

Jäger R, Mohr AE, Carpenter KC, International Society of Sports Nutrition Position Stand: Probiotics Journal of the International Society of Sports Nutrition (2019) 16:62

Jagim AR, Camic CL, Kisiolek J, Luedke J, Erickson J, Jones MT, Oliver JM.. Accuracy of Resting Metabolic Rate Prediction Equations in Athletes. J Strength Cond Res. 2018 Jul;32(7):1875-1881

Janssens, Y.; Nielandt, J.; Bronselaer, A.; Debunne, N.; Verbeke, F.; Wynendaele, E.; Van Immerseel, F.; Vandewynckel, Y.-P.; De Tré, G.; De Spiegeleer, B. Disbiome database: Linking the microbiome to disease. BMC Microbiol. 2018, 18, 50.

Jeukendrup AE, Vet-Joop K, Sturk A, et al. Relationship between gastro- intestinal complaints and endotoxaemia, cytokine release and the acute- phase reaction during and after a long-distance triathlon in highly trained men. Clin Sci (Lond). 2000;98:47–55.

Karl, J.P.; Margolis, L.M.; Madslien, E.H.; Murphy, N.E.; Castellani, J.W.; Gundersen, Y.; Hoke, A.V.; Levangie, M.W.; Kumar, R.; Chakraborty, N.; et al. Changes in intestinal microbiota composition and metabolism coincide with increased intestinal permeability in young adults under prolonged physiological stress. Am. J. Physiol. Gastrointest. Liver Physiol. 2017, 312, G559–G571.

Kay CD, Pereira-Caro G, Ludwig IA, Clifford MN, Crozier A. Anthocyanins and flavanones are more bioavailable than previously perceived: A review of recent evidence. In: Doyle MP, Klaenhammer TR, editors. Annual Review of Food Science and Technology, Vol 8. Palo Alto, USA: Annual Review Inc; 2017. p. 155–80.

Kennedy DO, Scholey AB. A glucose-caffeine Fenergy drink_ ameliorates subjective and performance deficits during prolonged cognitive demand. Appetite. 2004;42(3):331–3

Keytel LR, Goedecke JH, Noakes TD, Hiiloskorpi H, Laukkanen R, van der Merwe L, Lambert EV. Prediction of energy expenditure from heart rate monitoring during submaximal exercise.J Sports Sci. 2005 Mar;23(3):289-97.

Kondo S, Tanisawa K, Suzuki K, Terada S, Higuchi M. Preexercise Carbohydrate Ingestion and Transient Hypoglycemia: Fasting versus Feeding. Med Sci Sports Exerc. 2019 Jan;51(1):168-173.

Kreider RB, Wilborn CD, Taylor L, Campbell B, Almada AL, Collins R, Cooke M, Earnest CP, Greenwood M, Kalman DS, Kerksick CM, Kleiner SM, Leutholtz B, Lopez H, Lowery LM, Mendel R, Smith A, Spano M, Wildman R, Willoughby DS, Ziegenfuss TN, Antonio J. Issn exercise & sports nutrition review: research & recommendations. J Int Soc Sports Nutr. 2010;7(1):7.

Leatherwood W.E.; Dragoo, J.L. Effect of airline travel on performance: A review of the literature. Br. J. Sports Med. 2013, 47, 561–567.

Loat CE, Rhodes EC. Jet-lag and human performance. Sports Med (Auckland, NZ) 1989;8:226–38.

Lukaszuk JM, Robertson RJ, Arch JE, et al. Effect of a defined lacto-ovo- vegetarian diet and oral creatine monohydrate supplementation on plasma creatine concentration. J Strength Cond Res 2005; 19: 735-740.

Luscombe J, Murray AD, Jenkins E, et al. A rapid review to identify physical activity accrued while playing golf. BMJ Open 2017;7:e018993

Lynch H ,Johnston C, Wharton C. Plant-Based Diets: Considerations for Environmental Impact, Protein Quality, and Exercise Performance. Nutrients 2018, 10, 1841

Mach, N.; Fuster-Botella, D. Endurance exercise and gut microbiota: A review. J. Sport Health Sci. 2017, 6, 179–197.

Manfredini R.; Manfredini, F.; Fersini, C.; Conconi, F. Circadian rhythms, athletic performance, and jet lag. Br. J. Sports Med. 1998, 32, 101–106.

Maughan R. J., Leiper Jb, Shirreffs Sm. Restoration of fluid balance after exercise-induced dehydration: effects of food and fluid intake. European Journal of Applied Physiology 73:317–325, 1996.

Maughan R. J., Leiper Jb. Effects of sodium content of ingested fluids on post-exercise rehydration in man. European Journal of Applied Physiology 71:311–319, 1995.

Maughan RJ, Shirreffs SM. Dehydration and rehydration in competative sport. Scand J Med Sci Sports. 2010 Oct;20 Suppl 3:40-7

McDermott BP, Anderson SA, Armstrong LE, Casa DJ, Cheuvront SN, Cooper L, Kenney WL, O'Connor FG, Roberts WO. National Athletic Trainers' Association Position

Statement: Fluid Replacement for the Physically Active. J Athl Train. 2017 Sep;52(9):877-895.

McDermott, B.P. Anderson, S.A. Armstrong, L.E., Casa, D.J. Cheuvront, S.N.; Cooper, L.; Kenney, W.L.; O'Connor, F.G.; Roberts, W.O. National Athletic Trainers' Association Position Statement: Fluid Replacement for the Physically Active. J. Athl. Train. 2017, 52, 877–895.

Melina V., Craig W, Levin S (2016). Position of the academy of nutrition and dietetics: vegetarian diets. J. Acad. Nutr. Diet. 116:1970-1980

Moon JR. Body Composition in Athletes and Sports Nutrition: An Examination of the Bioimpedance Analysis Technique. Eur J Clin Nutr. 2013 Jan;67 Suppl 1:S54-9

Moore DR et al. Ingested protein dose response of muscle and albumin protein synthesis after resistance exercise in young man Am J Clin Nutr 2009;89:161-168.

Mumford PW1, Tribby AC, Poole CN, Dalbo VJ, Scanlan AT, Moon JR, Roberts MD, Young KC.Effect of Caffeine on Golf Performance and Fatigue during a Competitive Tournament. Med Sci Sports Exerc. 2016 Jan;48(1):132-8

Murray B, Rosenbloom. Fundamentals of glycogen metabolism for coaches and athletes. C. Nutr Rev. 2018 Apr 1;76(4):243-259.

Nieman D.C. (1988). Vegetarian dietary practices and endurance performance. Am. J. Clin. Nutr. 48 (Suppl):754-761

Nieman DC. Physical fitness and vegetarian diets: Is there a relation? Am J Clin Nutr 1999; 70(3 Suppl): 570S-575S.

Ørtenblad N, Westerblad H, Nielsen J. Muscle glycogen stores and fatigue. J Physiol. 2013 Sep 15;591(18):4405-13

Peukhuri K.; Sihvola, N.; Korpela, R. Diet promotes sleep duration and quality. Nutr. Res. 2012, 32, 309–319.

Phillips SM, Van Loon LJ. Dietary protein for athletes: from requirements to optimum adaptation. J Sports Sci 2011; 29-1: 29-38

Phillips SM. A brief review of higher dietary protein diets in weight loss: a focus on athletes. Sports Med. 2014;44(Suppl 2):S149–53.

Phillips SM. Fabbisogno proteico e integrazione negli sport di forza. Nutrizione. 2004; 20: 689-95.

Philpott JD, Witard OC, Galloway SDR. Applications of omega-3 polyunsaturated fatty acid supplementation for sport performance..Res Sports Med. 2019 27(2):219-237.

Racinais S.; Alonso, J.M.; Coutts, A.J.; Flouris, A.D.; Girard, O.; Gonzalez-Alonso, J.; Hausswirth, C.; Jay, O.; Lee, J.K.; Mitchell, N.; et al. Consensus recommendations on training and competing in the heat. Br. J. Sports Med. 2015, 49, 1164–1173

Ramos, C.L.; Thorsen, L.; Schwan, R.F.; Jespersen, L. Strain-specific probiotics properties of Lactobacillus fermentum, Lactobacillus plantarum and Lactobacillus brevis isolates from Brazilian food products. Food Microbiol. 2013, 36, 22–29

Reilly T, Waterhouse J, Burke LM, et al. Nutrition for travel. J Sports Sci 2007;25 (Suppl 1):S125–34.

Reilly T. Ergonomics in Sport and Physical Activity: Enhancing Performance and Improving Safety, 1st ed.; Human Kinetics: Champaign, IL, USA, 2010; pp. 75–95.

Reilly T. The body clock and athletic performance. Bioll Rhythm Res 2009;40:37–44.

Reilly T.; Waterhouse, J. Sports performance: Is there evidence that the body clock plays a role? Eur. J. Appl. Physiol. 2009, 106, 321–332.

Reilly T.; Waterhouse, J.; Edwards, B. Jet lag and air travel: Implications for performance. Clin. Sports Med. 2005, 24, 367–380.

Rodriguez NR, Di Marco NM, Langley S et al. American College of Sports Medicine position stand: nutrition and athletic performance. Med Sci Sports Exerc 2009: 41(3); 709-731

Rogerson D. Vegan diets: practical advice for athletes and exercisers ournal of the International Society of Sports Nutrition (2017) 14:36

Roza AM, Shizgal HM (1984). "The Harris Benedict equation reevaluated: resting energy requirements and the body cell mass" (PDF). The American Journal of Clinical Nutrition. 40 (1): 168–182

Ryan-Harshman M, Aldoori W. Vitamin B12 and health. Can Fam Physician 2008; 54: 536-54

Sanders SW, Moore JG. Gastrointestinal chronopharmacology: physiology, pharmacology and therapeutic implications. Pharmacol Ther 1992;54:1–15.

Santosa, S.; Farnworth, E.; Jones, P.J. Probiotics and their potential health claims. Nutr. Rev. 2006, 64, 265–274

Sawka M. N., Coyle EF. Influence of body water and blood volume on thermoregulation and exercise performance in the heat. Exerc. Sport Sci. Rev. 27:167–218, 1999.

Seeram NP, Zhang Y, McKeever R, Henning SM, Lee RP, Suchard MA, et al. Pomegranate juice and extracts provide similar levels of plasma and urinary ellagitannin metabolites in human subjects. J Med Food. 2008;11(2):390–4.

Shirreffs S. M., Maughan RJ. Volume repletion after exercise-induced volume depletion in humans: replacement of water and sodium losses. Am. J. Physiol. 274:F868–F875, 1998

Shona L. Halson T. Sleep in Elite Athletes and Nutritional Interventions to Enhance Sleep. Sports Med (2014) 44 (Suppl 1):S13–S23

Smit H, Rogers P. Effects of low doses of caffeine on cognitive performance, mood and thirst in low and higher caffeine consumers. Psychopharmacology (Berl). 2000;152(2):167–73.

Stauch M, Liu Y, Giesler M, et al. Physical activity level during a round of golf on a hilly course. J Sports Med Phys Fitness 1999;39:321–7.

Steenland K.; Deddens, J.A. Effect of travel and rest on performance of professional basketball players. Sleep 1997, 20, 366–369.

Tahara, Y.; Shibata, S. Chrono-biology, Chrono-pharmacology and Chrono-nutrition. J. Pharmacol. Sci. 2014, 124, 320–335. Saper, C.B.; Scammell, T.E.; Lu, J. Hypothalamic regulation of sleep and circadian rhythms. Nature 2005, 437, 1257–1263.

Tarnopolsky MA, Gibala M, Jeukendrup AE, Phillips SM. Nutritional Needs Of Elite Endurance Athletes. Part I: Carbohydrate And Fluid Requirements. Eur J Sport Sci. 2005;5(1):3–14.

Thomas DT, Erdman KA, Burke L. .J Position of the Academy of Nutrition and Dietetics, Dietitians of Canada, and the American College of Sports Medicine: Nutrition and Athletic Performance. .Acad Nutr Diet. 2016 Mar;116(3):501-528

Thomas DT, Erdman KA, Burke LM American College of Sports Medicine Joint Position Statement. Nutrition and Athletic Performance. Med Sci Sports Exerc. 2016 Mar;48(3):543-68.

Venderley AM, Campbell WW. Vegetarian diets: Nutritional considerations for athletes. Sports Med 2006; 36: 293-305

Venter R.E. Role of sleep in performance and recovery of athletes: A review article. South Afr. J. Res. Sport Phys. Educ. Recreat. 2012, 34, 167–184.
Vitale K, Getzin A Nutrition and Supplement Update for the Endurance Athlete: Review and Recommendations. Nutrients. 2019 Jun 7;11(6)

Wilkinson SB et al., Consumption of fluid skim milk promotes greater protein accretion after resistance exercise than does consuption of an isonitrogenous and isoenergetic soy-protein beverage Am J Clin Nutr 2007; 85 (4): 1031-1040.

Williams MH, Branch JD. Creatine supplementation and exercise performance: An update. J Am Coll Nutr 1998; 17: 216-234

Woo KS, Kwok CYT, Celermajer DS. Vegan diet, subnormal vitamin B-12 status and cardiovascular health. Nutrients. 2014;6(8):3259–73.

Woolf K, Manore MM. B-vitamins and exercise: Does exercise alter requirements? Int J Sport Nutr Exerc Metab 2006; 16: 453-484.

Wosinska L, Cotter PD, O'Sullivan O,* Guinane C The Potential Impact of Probiotics on the Gut Microbiome of Athletes Nutrients 2019, 11, 2270

Youngstedt S.D.; O'connor, P.J. The influence of air travel on athletic performance. Sports Med. 1999, SEP 28, 197–207.

Zouhal H, Jacob C, Delamarche P, Gratas-Delamarche. Catecholamines and the effects of exercise, training and gender. A Sports Med. 2008;38(5):401-23.

Zunzer SC, von Duvillard SP, Tschakert G, et al. Energy expenditure and sex differences of golf playing. J Sports Sci 2013;31:1045–53.

Printed in Great Britain
by Amazon